Brain Imaging in Psychiatry

CLINICAL INSIGHTS

Brain Imaging in Psychiatry

Edited by
JOHN M. MORIHISA, MD

Chief,
Clinical Neurophysiology Unit,
National Institute of Mental Health

AMERICAN PSYCHIATRIC PRESS, INC.
Washington, D.C.

© 1984 American Psychiatric Association

Library of Congress Cataloging in Publication Data

Main entry under title:

Brain imaging in psychiatry

(Clinical insights)
Includes bibliographies.
1. Brain—Radiography. 2. Neuropsychiatry. 3. Tomography. 4. Imaging systems in medicine. I. Morihisa, John M. II. Series.
RC386.6.T64B73   1984   616.89′07575   84-6303
ISBN 0-88048-052-1(pbk.)

Printed in the U.S.A.

Contents

5 Brain Electrical Activity Mapping (BEAM) in Psychiatry   77

John M. Morihisa, MD
Frank H. Duffy, MD
Richard Jed Wyatt, MD

Contributors

KAREN FAITH BERMAN, MD
Clinical Neuropsychiatry and Neurobehavior Section,
National Institute of Mental Health

MONTE S. BUCHSBAUM, MD
Professor, Department of Psychiatry and International Institute on
Brain and Behavior, Visual Imaging Center, University of California at Irvine

FRANK H. DUFFY, MD
Associate Professor, Department of Neurology, Harvard Medical School

RAQUEL E. GUR, MD, PhD
Director of Neuropsychiatry, Department of Psychiatry,
University of Pennsylvania

JOHN M. MORIHISA, MD
Chief, Clinical Neurophysiology Unit, National Institute of Mental Health

ISAK PROHOVNIK, PhD
Director, rCBF Laboratory, Department of Psychiatry,
College of Physicians and Surgeons, Columbia University

DANIEL R. WEINBERGER, MD
Chief, Clinical Neuropsychiatry and Neurobehavior Section,
and Director, rCBF Laboratory, National Institute of Mental Health

RICHARD JED WYATT, MD
Chief, Adult Psychiatry Branch, National Institute of Mental Health

RONALD F. ZEC, PhD
Clinical Neuropsychiatry and Neurobehavior Section,
National Institute of Mental Health

Introduction

During the past five years a number of remarkable new techniques for visualizing brain function have been introduced to medical research. These approaches employ high-speed computers, color graphics, and sophisticated software to detect patterns from limited laboratory clues. Computerized axial tomography (the "CT" scan) has revolutionized medical diagnosis and treatment by providing a three-dimensional view of the body. Psychiatry is now exploring the use of such technology in the study of mental illness. Like other new techniques, these have potential limitations as well as benefits. The benefits may be new clinical procedures for diagnosis and treatment. Potential limitations include the misinterpretation of data, an overdependence on automated analysis, and prematurely drawing conclusions or rejecting techniques. The purpose of this book is to describe brain-imaging techniques now applied in psychiatry, to clarify the theory behind them and the problems in interpreting their results, and to provide a framework to judge their potential usefulness. The chapters in this book were originally presented as part of a symposium on brain imaging at the Annual Meeting of the American Psychiatric Association, May 11, 1983.

In this monograph we discuss three brain-imaging methods: regional cerebral blood flow (rCBF), positron emission tomography

(PET) and brain electrical activity mapping (BEAM). Case studies present the theory, applications, and recent findings of these brain-imaging techniques.

In the first chapter, Buchsbaum introduces one of the imaging techniques most recently applied to psychiatric questions, PET. In his discussion, theory, clinical applications, and recent findings in schizophrenia and affective illness are reported that suggest frontal lobe hypometabolism is related to these conditions. However, it is noted that the use of PET in psychiatry is still in its infancy.

The following three chapters are devoted to one of the forms of brain imaging longest used in psychiatry, that of regional cerebral blood flow (rCBF). The first of these chapters addresses the theory and limitations of the technique, the second its applications in research, the last focuses on its use in the study of schizophrenia.

Prohovnik presents a short but comprehensive review of the theoretical basis of rCBF, with attention to issues of methodology. This chapter should allow the reader to understand rCBF and to evaluate reports in the literature. Prohovnik uses examples to demonstrate some of the problems in interpreting rCBF studies. Finally, he emphasizes the potential value of "activation" rCBF measurements, in which the subject performs a cognitive task.

Berman and Weinberger present the practical problems in applying this theory to investigating specific clinical phenomena. They describe testing patients who have specific neuroanatomical damage to provide biological validation of the rCBF system. They also describe the research strategy presently employed in studying schizophrenia, which again underscores the value of "activation" rCBF studies.

Finally, Gur reports a study of patients that shows the importance of controlling for the effects of sex and medication in rCBF research. She agrees with Prohovnik that studies of the resting state have significant limitations. Gur uses cognitive activation tasks to reveal abnormalities in hemispheric lateralization. Her results support her hypothesis of left hemispheric overactivation in schizophrenics.

In the last chapter we describe a new brain-imaging technique designed to analyze and present graphically electroencephalographic features of mental illness. This technique creates color maps of brain electrical activity, maps which suggest that the frontal lobes and left parietal region are sites of abnormal physiology that may be relevant to understanding schizophrenia. This chapter considers together the findings of a variety of brain-imaging techniques, but cautions that apparent correlations in their findings should be used to guide future investigations rather than be taken as conclusive results. In fact, we point out that the findings of recent rCBF work reported here disagree with those of the first rCBF studies of schizophrenia. Some of the weaknesses inherent in these techniques are reviewed and a hypothesis is proposed about left hemispheric abnormalities in schizophrenia. The volume concludes by suggesting that the various imaging techniques should be used to complement each other, thereby increasing our chance of clarifying abnormalities of brain function in mental illness.

John M. Morihisa, M.D.

(*NOTE:* The work described in Chapter 2 was supported in part by NIMH grant MH35636; the work described in Chapter 4 was supported in part by NIMH grant MH30456.)

1

Positron Emission Tomography (PET) in Psychiatry

Monte S. Buchsbaum, M.D.

1

Positron Emission Tomography (PET) in Psychiatry

In the past our approach to the brain has been necessarily indirect, employing peripheral fluids to assess central and regional neurochemical processes. Blood, urine, skin and muscle biopsy, and cerebrospinal fluid are valuable reflectors of the neurochemical and neuropharmacological activity of the brain, but are removed in time and place from disordered thought processes and diluted by the products of both functional and dysfunctional brain systems. Biopsy studies have helped in studying the functional disorders of organs like the liver, but they are destructive to the brain and less useful because unlike these organs, the brain has a regional variation in its chemistry. The experimental insights from animal studies focusing on the pharmacology of individual cell groups—in striatum or locus coeruleus, for example—cannot easily or unambiguously be applied to clinical populations. Positron emission tomography (PET) is a versatile approach utilizing the mathematics of x-ray transmission scanning (CT scanning) to produce slice images of radioisotope distribution (Brownell et al. 1982). PET makes possible a wide range of metabolic studies. Positron emitters such as carbon-11 or fluorine-18 can be used to label glucose, amino acids, drugs, neurotransmitter precursors, and many other molecules and examine their distribution and fate in discrete cell groups.

ASSESSING REGIONAL FUNCTION BY BLOOD FLOW

The major energy source for the brain is glucose, and its use is closely related to local functional activity, oxygen consumption, and blood flow (Sokoloff 1981). This coupling holds not only for generalized brain states, as in coma or excitement, but also is a localized mechanism affecting small brain areas. Before the development of PET techniques, cerebral blood flow, together with the electroencephalogram, were the principal measures of regional brain function in clinical studies. In early research, Kety et al. (1948) studied the cerebral blood flow correlates of schizophrenia with their nitrous oxide technique for the whole brain. They found no differences between their 22 patients and normal controls, but noted: "There remains the possibility that local disturbances confined to small but important regions may still occur since the method used yields only mean values for the entire brain."

Ingvar and Franzen (1974) measured cerebral blood flow in 31 schizophrenic patients and 10 neurologically normal male alcoholics. They used intra-arterial xenon injection and 32 detectors to evaluate cortical flow. Subjects were tested at rest, usually with their eyes closed. Control subjects had relatively higher frontal than posterior blood flow while schizophrenic patients had low frontal flow, especially those patients with symptoms of indifference, inactivity, and autism. Flow increases in postcentral temporal-occipital and parietal regions were associated with symptoms of disturbed cognition. Chronic schizophrenics also showed smaller increases in frontal blood flow with simple tasks. In highly disturbed patients, the task of naming objects in pictures produced slight and insignificant increases in frontal flow (Franzen and Ingvar 1975). Controls showed large increases, although they performed a somewhat more difficult task (Raven's Matrices), which might have contributed to this effect. Postcentral flow increased about equally in both groups, which supports the hypothesis of hypofrontal function in schizophrenia.

Ingvar and Philipson (1977) measured blood flow in the frontal lobes in studies of "motor ideation." They mapped regional blood flow in subjects at rest, as the subjects imagined a slow rhythmic clenching of the right hand, and as they made actual hand movements. At rest, these subjects had higher flow in frontal than in postcentral regions. When they imagined hand movements, flow increased in premotor frontal regions, especially in superior frontal, inferior frontal, and temporal pole regions.

Mathew and colleagues (1980, 1981) studied cerebral blood flow in patients with schizophrenia and depression using inhalation of xenon-133. They found schizophrenics showed decreased blood flow in the whole right hemisphere while patients with depression showed decreased blood flow in the whole left hemisphere. Controls showed higher right frontal than occipital values (frontal to occipital ratio, 1.05) than did schizophrenics (ratio, 1.00), but this difference did not reach statistical significance.

Ariel et al. (1983) found normal and schizophrenics to have significant differences in anteroposterior blood flow. It is important to note that high individual differences in regional blood flow make within-subject regional comparisons, such as ratios, a critical test of the hypotheses.

PET METHODS

The measurement of blood flow by xenon-133 washout, like rheoencephalography and electroencephalography, is essentially a two-dimensional technique. Flow values in the gray matter of the cortex or underlying white matter are assessed and plotted on a two-dimensional projection of the cortical surface. PET is a three-dimensional technique, developing consecutive slice images and assessing each cubic centimeter of brain tissue. The development of PET scanning technology is well reviewed by Phelps et al. (1982). The distribution of an extensive variety of positron-emitting radiopharmaceuticals can be determined using the mathematics of computed tomography.

What molecules should psychiatry study? The therapeutic success of neuroleptics suggests that their binding sites should be studied. Ingvar's (1980) findings suggest the dynamic imaging of blood flow or local metabolism. These two types of PET imaging are only the beginning of new approaches to studying various problems in psychiatry and human behavior.

IMAGING OF RECEPTORS

Neuroleptics have a higher binding affinity for the dopaminergic receptors in the brain than for other receptors. Thus, when labeled for PET analysis, a drug like chlorpromazine might reveal the location and density of dopamine receptors. The PET scans could reflect the number of receptors per unit volume, receptor affinity for the labeled compound, and the concentrations of natural receptor agonists available. PET dynamically reflects the neurochemical status of the dopamine system at the time of the scan. Unfortunately, other factors can also affect labeling. Neuroleptic ligands bind to receptors other than the dopamine receptor. The presence of dopamine receptors with different affinities complicates the direct interpretation of the quantitative image. Metabolic products of neuroleptics that retain the positron-emitting isotope would appear, although perhaps with a time course slower than the half-life of the isotope (Comar et al. 1979). In addition, these drugs are lipid-soluble and enter myelin and fatty material. The image reflects all of these influences.

The first clinical PET study of neuroleptics tested carbon-11-labeled chlorpromazine in 22 schizophrenic patients who had not taken neuroleptics for several months (Comar et al. 1979). The images obtained in this study were not entirely dissimilar to those obtained with glucose, with gray matter labeled more strongly than white. The cerebellum, where dopaminergic receptors are not thought to occur, appears clearly; this indicates relatively high nonspecific binding. Recently, Wagner et al. (1983) used carbon-11-labeled methylspiperone in a PET study on one normal volunteer. This tracer bound more selectively to caudate than to cerebellum (with a 4.4:1 ratio at 70 to 130 min). This method may prove powerful in demonstrating receptor abnormalities in schizophrenics. Another recent study with fluorine-18-labeled L-dopa also showed caudate and frontal cortex concentraion, demonstrating the versatility of PET in studying dopamine neurochemistry in man.

BLOOD FLOW

Blood flow can be measured with a number of tracers, including krypton-77, oxygen-15-labeled water, $^{13}NH_3$, and molecules labeled with fluorine-18 (Phelps et al. 1982). The short half-lives of oxygen-15 and $^{13}N_3$ (2 and 10 min) make them suitable for behavioral studies using a series of scans to compare different psychological tasks over 30 minutes to 2 hours. Ingvar and Philipson (1977) found large changes in blood flow with mental activity, with many brain areas showing a change in flow of more than 50 percent, and found also that schizophrenics may show differences in these dynamic shifts. The rigorous testing of any of the major psychological theories of schizophrenia, such as the theory of selective attentional deficit, requires at least two scans of a patient, one while the patient is doing the attentional task and a contrasting control. Since most experimental tasks in schizophrenia research have motor, perceptual, and cognitive phases, many scan studies will be needed to compare the components of the tasks in normal controls to characterize the nature of the deficit. One possible disadvantage of the very short half-life flow studies with ^{15}O and ^{13}N is that the isotope administration and scanning must both take place in less than 10 minutes. The subject must perform the psychological task in the scanner room and then be positioned and scanned. With some kinetic models, scanning must actually be done during the task (see the discussion in Phelps et al. 1982), making complete sensory control and stimulus administration difficult. The short-lived isotopes used in these studies must also be produced by a cyclotron on site.

GLUCOSE METABOLIC RATE

PET imaging of glucose metabolic rate rather than of blood flow has both advantages and disadvantages for psychiatric studies. The

Sokoloff technique (1982) uses a fluorine-18-labeled analogue of glucose, 2-deoxyglucose (FDG).

FDG is taken up by the brain much as glucose itself. But glucose is rapidly metabolized to CO_2 and H_2O. Since CO_2 is a gas it diffuses rapidly across tissues impeding high-resolution images and precise quantification of metabolic rates. The unusual structure of 2-deoxyglucose allows its metabolism in the first step in the glycolytic pathway (to 2-deoxyglucose-6-phosphate), but no further. Since its metabolism stops at this point, the cells are labeled accordingly in proportion to their glucose uptake. After injection, FDG is almost entirely taken up over the next 30 to 40 minutes, most of it in the first 10. This can be done in a separate and psychologically controlled environment. The scan begun at 50 minutes thus reflects glucose use during the initial controlled period after injection, not during the scan operation (Figures 1–3), which allows study of psychophysical tasks, directed interviews about emotional subjects, or even REM sleep (Figures 4 and 5). The need for the subject to sustain the activity for 30 minutes limits the temporal resolution of the study, however, and the habituated response to sensory stimulation could predominate in the image of glucose use. Nevertheless, FDG has been the tracer predominantly used in psychiatric studies to date.

TOMOGRAPHIC MAPPING OF GLUCOSE USE DURING SENSORY STIMULATION

As blood flow is sensitive to psychological tasks, local glucose use is highly sensitive to sensory stimulation. Visual stimulation in one hemifield is associated with increases in glucose use in the contralateral visual cortex (Greenberg et al. 1981), and more glucose is used when two eyes are stimulated than when one eye is stimulated (Phelps et al. 1981a). As visual stimulation is increased—from having the subject keep eyes closed to presenting simple white light, then a checkerboard pattern reversal, and finally having the subject view a park outside the laboratory, the use of glucose by visual cortex increases up to twofold (Phelps et al. 1981a, 1981b). Somatosensory and auditory stimulation also in-

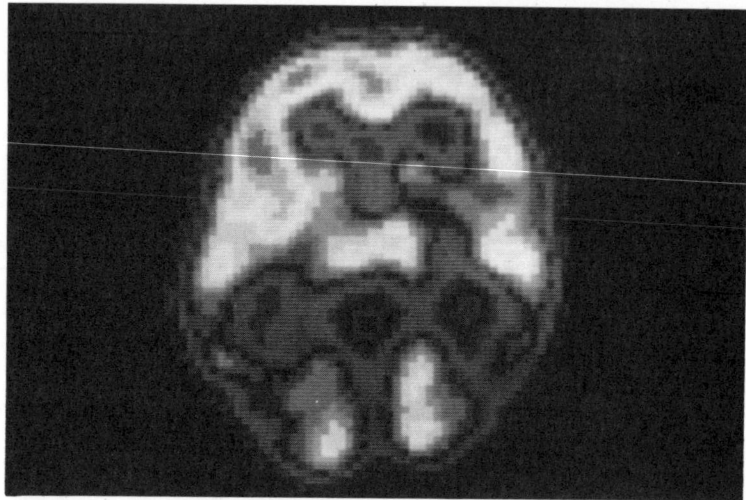

Figure 1. Normal control PET scan with FDG. Shown is a horizontal slice about 40 mm above the canthomeatal line (the line joining the outer canthus of the eye and the external auditory meatus). This normal volunteer received shock stimuli during the FDG uptake while resting with his eyes closed. Note that primary visual regions (bottom of slice) are relatively inactive whereas the thalamus (center of the slice) and frontal lobes are quite active.

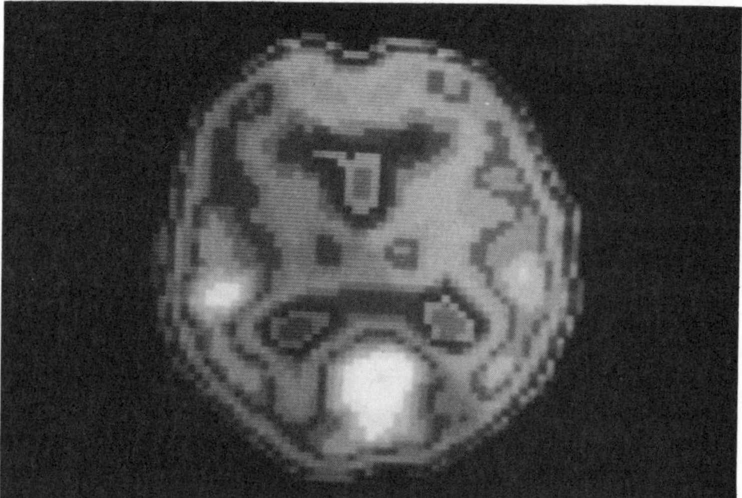

Figure 2. PET scan of patient with bipolar affective disorder under the same shock condition as the normal control in Figure 1. Frontal lobes and thalamus are both much less active relative to visual areas than in normal control.

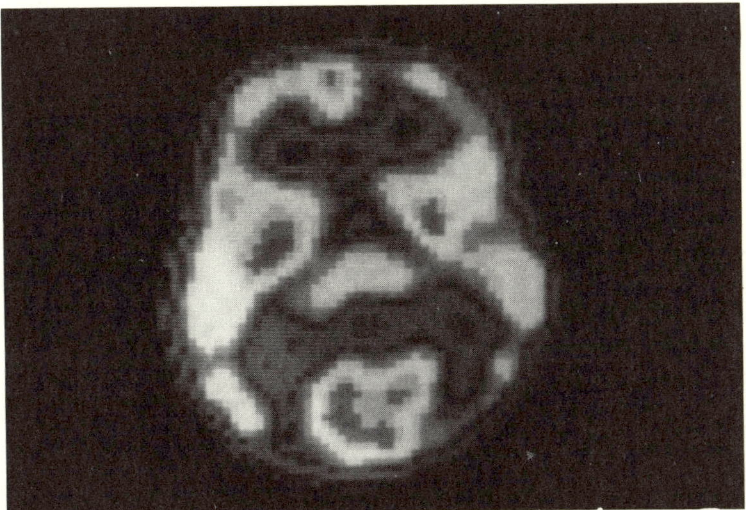

Figure 3. PET scan of a patient with schizophrenia. Here, visual area shows high metabolic rate (compare with Figure 1). Frontal lobes show relatively lower activity with a gap just right of center in the frontal area.

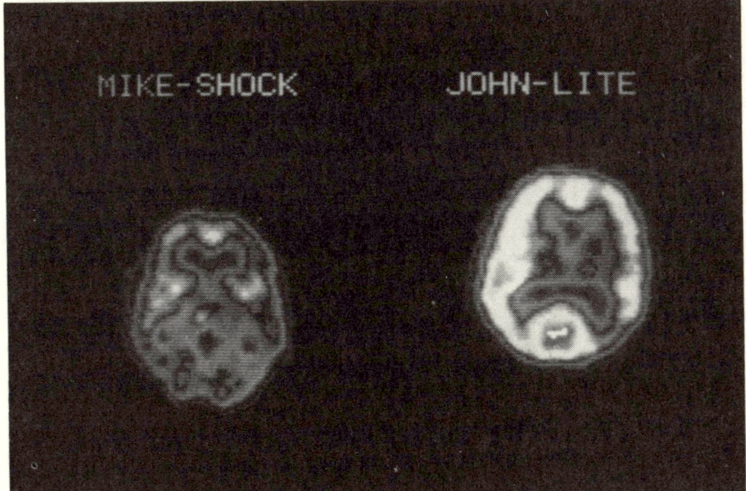

Figure 4. The effect of performing a task on PET is shown in scans of normal identical twins. During FDG uptake, Mike received a series of brief electrical stimuli to his right forearm. John did a standard visual vigilance test. Note increased glucose metabolic in visual cortex of John compared to Mike.

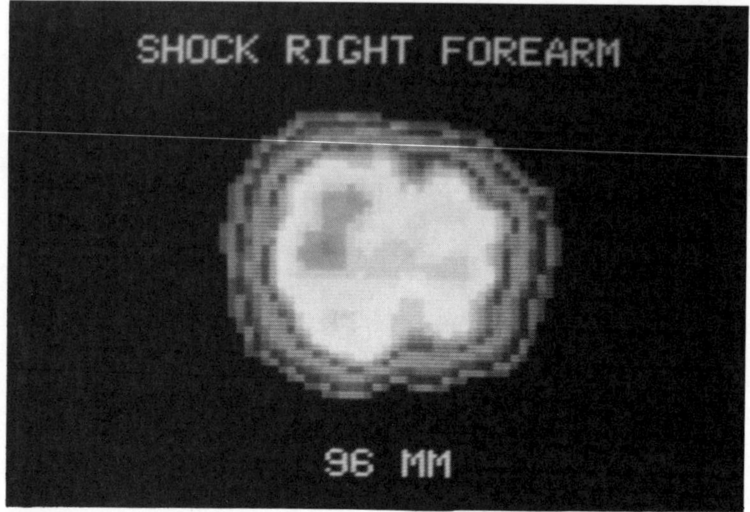

Figure 5. Effect of right forearm electrical stimulation on left pre- and postcentral cortex.

crease glucose use in the primary sensory areas (Greenberg et al. 1981). Electrical stimulation of the right forearm has been associated with greater glucose use in the left than the right postcentral, but not precentral, gyrus (Buchsbaum et al. 1983). Phelps et al. (1981b) reported that whole brain glucose use was little changed by visual stimulation. Along with the results of Ingvar and Philipson (1977) all these findings suggest that control of sensory stimulation and mental activity is critical for reliable and interpretable results in studying psychiatric patients.

PET STUDIES OF PATIENTS WITH SCHIZOPHRENIA

Farkas et al. (1980) studied a 45-year-old patient with a history of schizophrenia since the age of 16. This patient had taken no neuroleptic medication before the scan. The patient showed a 40 percent depression in frontal glucose use compared to an unspecified control population. A second scan obtained when the patient was on phenothiazines showed an apparent return toward normal. These researchers also noted a relative decrease in glucose use in the left hemisphere, especially in temporal and motor cortex.

The hypofrontal pattern of glucose use seen by Farkas et al. (1980) parallels the findings about blood flow of Ingvar and coworkers. This case report of hypofrontality is consistent with the findings of a later preliminary report on more patients (Farkas et al. 1981). Details about patients' drug dosage, ages, and sex distribution, and about the statistical analysis used are not available at this writing.

We recently reported (Buchsbaum et al. 1982a) on local cerebral uptake of fluorine-18-labeled 2-fluoro-2-deoxy-D-glucose (2^{18}FDG) in eight unmedicated schizophrenic patients and in six age-matched normal volunteers, as measured by PET. Subjects sat resting with eyes closed in an acoustically controlled, darkened room following injection of 3 to 5 mCi of FDG. Following uptake of FDG, we obtained seven to eight horizontal brain scans parallel to the canthomeatal line (a line connecting the outer canthus of the eye with the external auditory meatus). Scans were treated digitally, with a 2-cm strip peeled off each slice and ratios to whole slice activity computed. Patients with schizophrenia showed lower ratios in frontal cortex, indicating relatively lower glucose use in this region than in normal controls; this was consistent with previously reported studies of regional cerebral blood flow. No clear evidence of left-right differences was found in the cortex. Patients also showed diminished ratios for a 2-cm square positioned over central gray matter areas on the left, but not the right, side (a region including the anterior thalamus, caudate, globus pallidus, internal capsule, and part of the ventricles).

In this study of glucose metabolism, we chose that subjects be in the resting state with eyes closed in order to compare our data directly with studies of blood flow (Ingvar and Franzen 1974; Ingvar 1980). These studies found lower frontal flow in schizophrenic patients and did not compare both hemispheres. Thus, the absence of cortical asymmetries, especially in normals, is not altogether unexpected. Subjects were merely instructed to rest with their eyes closed for 30 minutes, an entirely unstructured task with no clear hemispheric assignment.

Our second group of patients received somatosensory stimulation to the right forearm. Ingvar (1980) had noted that frontal blood flow increased in subjects who put their hands in ice water, but less so in schizophrenics. This finding was consistent with observations by ourselves and others (Davis et al. 1979a; Davis and Buchsbaum 1981) of diminished sensitivity to pain in schizophrenics (Buchsbaum et al. 1980; Davis et al. 1979b). We anticipated that, in addition to possibly enhanced hypofrontality, we might observe in schizophrenics some lateralized indication of affective response to pain.

In this second series of experiments we studied 16 schizophrenic patients and 11 patients with bipolar affective disorder as controls. Patients were unmedicated at least 14 days and an average of 39.8 days before the procedure. They were then administered FDG just before receiving a series of unpleasant electrical stimuli to their right forearms, one every second for 34 minutes while resting with their eyes closed in a darkened, acoustically controlled chamber. Following monitored stimulation in the controlled environment, subjects were scanned and resulting images were converted to values of glucose use in micromoles/100 g/min according to Sokoloff's model. Data were analyzed with a 4-way ANOVA with independent groups (normals, schizophrenics, and those with affective disorders) and repeated measures for slice level (supra-, mid-, and infraventricular), hemisphere (right, left), and anteroposterior position (four sectors). Normals and patients both showed a significant anteroposterior gradient in glucose use with highest values for the frontmost sector. Patients with schizophrenia and those with affective illness both showed less anteroposterior gradient, especially at superior levels, which was statistically confirmed by ANOVA. Absolute glucose levels in patients that were actually higher in posterior regions, rather than lower in frontal regions, were the largest contributors to the effect. No significant correlation was observed between ratios of anterior to posterior regions and length of time off neuroleptics, body weight, or gender.

PET studies of the well-known Genain quadruplets (Rosenthal 1963) similarly indicated relative hypofrontality. There were no statistically significant group differences in whole brain glucose use nor left-right asymmetries. These results are consistent with our earlier reports of relative hypofrontal function in schizophrenics compared with controls, and with the blood flow studies of Ingvar and Franzen (1974) and Ariel et al. (1983), as well as with the early findings of Kety et al. (1948) of no whole brain metabolic differences.

Artifacts of the effects of drugs on PET scans are another increasingly important issue as it becomes increasingly difficult to find patients who have never been treated with neuroleptics. Neuroleptics seem to decrease glucose use throughout the brain in autoradiographic studies of rats (McCulloch et al. 1982). Clinical studies of blood flow also seem to indicate that neuroleptics lower blood flow (Risberg 1980), perhaps in frontal regions especially, but specific statistical confirmation of this regional effect is lacking. The first patient of Farkas et al. (1980), however, who had never been treated with neuroleptics, showed responses similar to those of our subjects (Buchsbaum et al. 1982a) who had not taken medication for an average of 37.6 days.

Patients with schizophrenia and affective illness did not differ in anteroposterior ratios. The possibility of missing a true group difference was increased by the relatively small sample size, diagnostic heterogeneity within the affective disorder sample, mood heterogeneity, and the limited number of brain areas so far assessed. The lack of diagnostic specificity may well indicate that relative hypofrontality is a general feature of illness or hospitalization, familiarity with procedures, differences in anxiety in patients and controls, or other factors. However, other more extensively studied biological markers, including smooth pursuit eye movements, platelet monoamine oxidase and attentional deficits also show affective/schizophrenia overlap. All of these biological markers may well indicate some important communality between these two functional psychoses.

LATERAL RECONSTRUCTION OF PET

This analysis used the approximately-equal-area lateral-brain projection previously developed for electrophysiological topography

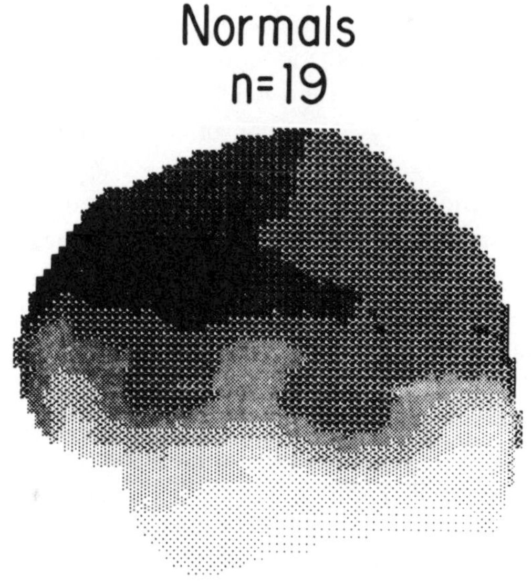

Figure 6. Group averages of left hemisphere lateral cerebral glucography shown for normal controls and patients with schizophrenia and affective disorder. Averages were computed pixel by pixel. Each side view has been normalized with every pixel in the side view expressed as the following quantity: (pixel value minus hemisphere mean)/hemisphere standard deviation. The scale for averages is standard deviation units. Note that patients showed a more posterior temporal pattern of relative activity while normals were significantly higher in frontal cortex.

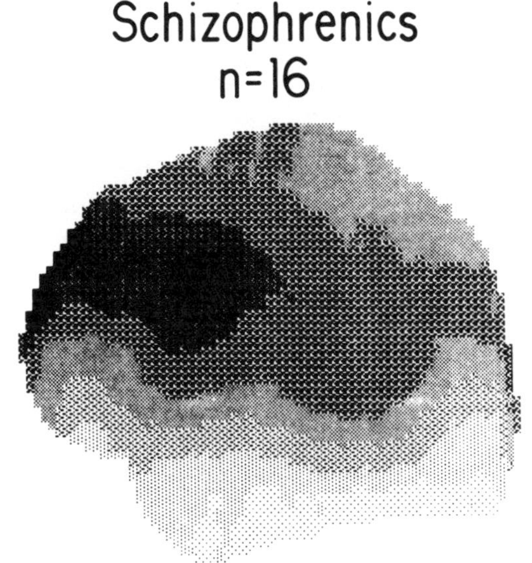
Schizophrenics
n=16

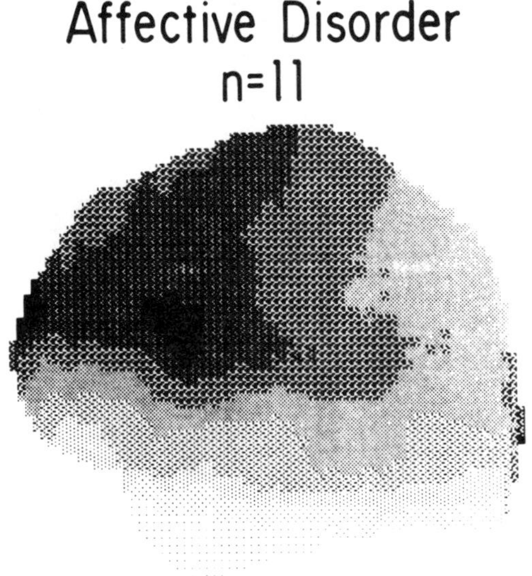
Affective Disorder
n=11

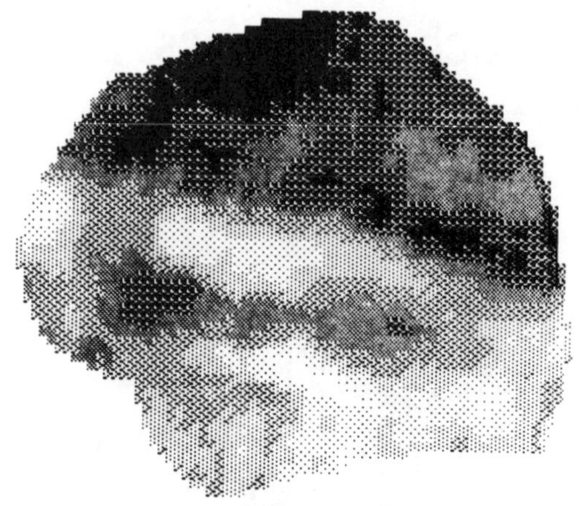

N vs. S

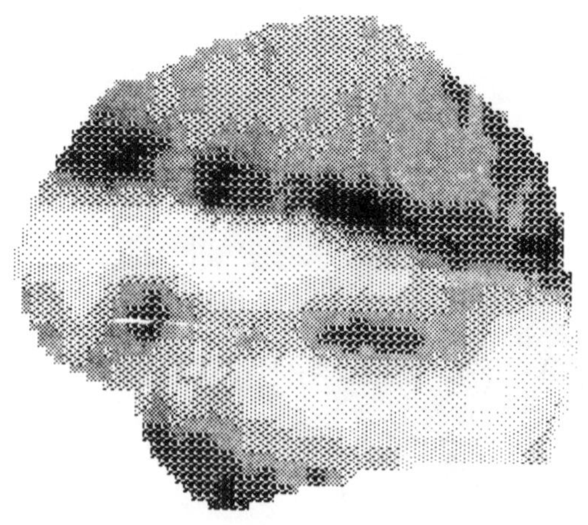

N vs. A

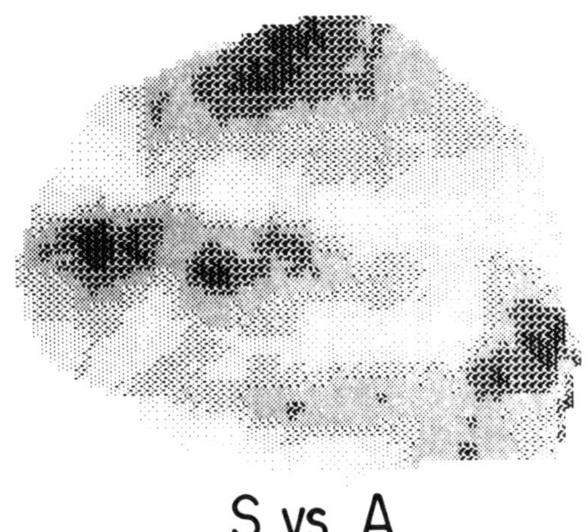

Figure 7. Statistical comparisons (t-tests) are shown for normal controls versus patients with schizophrenia (N vs. S), normal controls versus patients with affective disorder (N vs. A), and patients with schizophrenia versus patients with affective disorder (S vs. A). The t-tests were computed pixel by pixel. The scale for the t-tests is adjusted so that $p < 0.5$, two-tailed, is black (normals higher) or white (patients higher).

(Buchsbaum et al. 1982b). The cortical peel (the same one used to isolate sectors for the ANOVA) was extracted from each slice. A line joining each successive pixel on the outline to the center of the slice was calculated, and the values of all pixels in the peel traversed by this line were averaged; this averaging generated one mean cortical glucose value for each pixel in the slice outline. These series of glucose values were then scaled in length to fit the anteroposterior dimension of the lateral brain outline at the appropriate level.

Slice level was expressed in percentage of brain height, a calculation accomplished by identifying the slice level as a percentage of head height (measured perpendicular to the canthomeatal line to the top of the head) and translating this value to an approximate percentage of brain height using an atlas (Matsui and Hirano 1978). An interpolation routine next approximated pixel values between the slice levels.

This procedure has several features that make it suitable for studies of schizophrenia. First, its results can be directly compared with the two-dimensional data on cerebral blood flow previously obtained. Second, it allows the computation of mean glucose use images with pixel by pixel statistics, for exploratory analyses in group comparisons (Figures 6 and 7). Third, direct comparison of electrophysiological and glucographic topography becomes possible.

IMAGING MODALITIES TO SUPPLEMENT PET

Three new imaging techniques have appeared that complement and extend PET: nuclear magnetic resonance, single photon tomography, and electroencephalographic topography.

Nuclear Magnetic Resonance (NMR) Imaging

Nuclear magnetic resonance (NMR) imaging is based on reception of radiofrequencies emitted by nuclei of different elements in the brain following application of a magnetic field (Brownell et al. 1982; James et al. 1982). Using principles similar to those of X-ray CT scan reconstruction, NMR can provide a slice image. The first clinical use of NMR was to image the hydrogen nucleus, mostly in H_2O. This provides a picture of water distribution. Since gray and white matter differ significantly in water content, NMR can better distinguish the structures of gray matter than can CT scanning. CT scanning images x-ray transmission, which differs little between gray and white matter. No psychiatric studies have been done yet with NMR, but determining the size and shape of the basal ganglia and limbic structures are obvious targets of interest for studies of schizophrenia and affective illness.

NMR will make possible a detailed anatomic horizontal image to complement the functional PET images. FDG does not provide an anatomic image, only a functional one, which can lead to ambiguous interpretations. High metabolic activity in the region of the basal ganglia could be caudate in one group and putamen in another. NMR can provide a detailed atlas of gray and white matter for each subject to help interpret metabolic images.

The NMR technique has a potential for going beyond anatomic studies to measure other nuclei such as phosphorus (^{31}P) in cell energy metabolism and appropriately labeled pharmaceuticals. But the low concentrations of these nuclei make the production of high-resolution slice images currently unattainable. The use of stronger magnetic fields and other technical improvements will be necessary before NMR can yield such images.

Electroencephalographic (EEG) Imaging

The recording of brain waves has been used for years to detect tumors, epilepsy, and other brain diseases as well as to study psychological functioning. EEG patterns are exquisitely sensitive to the effects of drugs and can be used to predict the action or appropriate dosage of new drugs. The EEG can also be employed in collecting signals from electrodes placed over the entire scalp. When analyzed by spectral analysis, these signals yield amplitude measures for each of the major EEG frequency patterns—delta, alpha, and beta. A map of the electrical activity on the surface of the brain can be constructed by interpolating values between each observed point (Buchsbaum et al. 1982b). In initial studies, this method indicated frontal increases in delta activity (Morihisa et al.

1982; Buchsbaum et al. 1982c; Morihisa et al. 1983) in schizophrenic patients. This finding is consistent with the relative hypofrontality seen in blood flow studies and with PET, since increased delta activity has been associated with cerebrovascular deficits (Ingvar et al. 1976; Tolonen and Sulg 1981).

Using briefly presented words or tones and a computer technique known as averaging, an "evoked potential"—the specific brain response to the stimulus—can be recorded. Evoked potentials from scalp EEG leads spaced at 1 cm can reveal the sensory stations on the cortex corresponding to parts of the body as close together as wrist and finger. There are great possibilities for exploring the entire cortex of the brain with mapping techniques and for using them to better define neurophysiological and pharmacological effects. Preliminary data reveal decreases in the amplitude of evoked potentials, especially in parietal areas (Buchsbaum 1982d). With leads attached to a flexible helmet and rapid computer sampling, arrays of 64 to 128 leads can be used in clinical procedures.

Single Photon Tomography

While the most widely used noninvasive method of measuring cerebral blood flow has been the xenon-133 washout procedure, its use has been limited largely to studies of cortical surface. Recently, computed tomographic approaches have been developed that employ a rotating gamma camera.

A new radiopharmaceutical is now available, iodine-123-iodo-amphetamine (I-123-IMP), which is given intravenously and is taken up in the brain proportionally to blood flow (Lassen et al. 1983; Kuhl et al. 1982). Comparative studies show good correspondence between regional cerebral blood flow estimated by xenon-133 and by I-123-IMP. The advantage of I-123-IMP is that it is bound in the brain in a blood flow distribution for 30 to 45 minutes after injection, a time long enough to permit computed emission tomographic imaging using a rotating gamma camera. With this method, tomographic slices of the brain may be produced in axial, sagittal, coronal, or oblique projections.

Rush et al. (in press) used single photon tomography to study patients with affective disorders who had been free of psychoactive medications for at least seven days. Decreased blood flow was observed in patients with unipolar depression, consistent with the results of Mathew et al. (1980) and Silfverskiold et al. (in press). However, unlike the patients of Silfverskiold et al., patients in this study with manic or mixed-phase bipolar illness had higher flows than controls. Using a four-faced camera and xenon-133, Lassen et al. (1983) reported 1.7-cm full-width-half maximum resolution, which approaches that of the previous generation of PET scanners. The lower cost of single photon scanners and their use of longer lived isotopes than positron emitters make them desirable for the study of cerebral phenomena involving rather large cortical areas.

CONCLUSION

Although PET has many potential applications in psychiatric studies, psychiatry has only begun to explore the use of this technique. Technical advances in PET, along with related refinements in research strategies, will in time define its role in clinical psychiatry.

References

Ariel RN, Golden CJ, Berg PA, et al: Regional cerebral blood flow in schizophrenics. Arch Gen Psychiatry 40:258–263, 1983

Brownell GL, Budinger TF, Lauterbur PC, et al: Positron tomography and nuclear magnetic resonance imaging. Science 215:619–626, 1982

Buchsbaum MS, Davis GC, van Kammen DP: Diagnostic classification and the endorphin hypothesis of schizophrenia: individual differences and psychopharmacological strategies, in Perspectives in Schizophrenia Research. Edited by Baxter C, Melnechuk T. New York, Raven Press, 1980, pp 177–194

Buchsbaum MS, Ingvar DH, Kessler R, et al: Cerebral glucography with positron tomography. Arch Gen Psychiatry 39:251–259, 1982a

Buchsbaum MS, Rigal F, Coppola R, et al: A new system for gray-level surface distribution maps of electrical activity. Electroencephalogr Clin Neurophysiol 53:237–242, 1982b

Buchsbaum MS, Cappelletti J, Coppola R, et al: New methods to determine the CNS effects of antigeriatric compounds: EEG topography and glucose use. Drug Develoment Research 2:489–496, 1982c

Buchsbaum MS, King AC, Cappelletti J, et al: Visual evoked potential topography in patients with schizophrenia and normal controls. Advances in Biological Psychiatry 9:1–7, 1982d

Buchsbaum MS, Holcomb HH, Johnson J, et al: Cerebral metabolic consequences of electrical stimulation in normal individuals. Human Neurobiology 2:35–38, 1983

Comar D, Zarifian E, Verhas M, et al: Brain distribution and kinetics of 11C-chloropromazine in schizophrenics. Psychiatry Res 1:23–29, 1979

Davis GC, Buchsbaum MS: Pain sensitivity and endorphins in functional psychoses, in Modern Problems of Pharmacopsychiatry. Edited by Ban TA, et al. Basel, Switzerland, S. Karger, 1981, pp 99–108

Davis GC, Buchsbaum MS, van Kammen DP, et al: Analgesia to pain stimuli in schizophrenics reversed by naltrexone. Psychiatry Res 1:61–69, 1979a

Davis GC, Buchsbaum MS, Bunney WE Jr: Research in endorphins and schizophrenia. Schizophr Bull 5:244–250, 1979b

Farkas T, Reivich M, Alavi A, et al: The application of ^{18}F 2-deoxy-2-fluoro-D-glucose and positron emission tomography in the study of psychiatric conditions, in Cerebral Metabolism and Neural Function. Edited by Passonneau JV, Hawkins RA, Lust WD, et al. Baltimore, MD, Williams and Wilkins, 1980, pp 403–408

Farkas T, Wolff AP, Jaeger J, et al: Regional cerebral glucose utilization in chronic schizophrenia. Abstract presented at the Third World Congress of Biological Psychiatry, Stockholm, June 28–July 3, 1981

Franzen G, Ingvar DH: Absence of activation in frontal structures during psychological testing of chronic schizophrenics. J Neurol Neurosurg Psychiatry 38:1027–1032, 1975

Garnett ES, Firnau G, Nahmias C: Dopamine visualized in the basal ganglia of living man. Nature 305:137–138, 1983

Greenberg JH, Reivich M, Alavi A, et al: Metabolic mapping of functional activity in human subjects with the [^{18}F] fluoro-deoxyglucose technique. Science 212:678–680, 1981

Ingvar DH: Abnormal distribution of cerebral activity in chronic schizophrenia: a neurophysiological interpretation, in Perspectives in Schizophrenia Research. Edited by Baxter CF, Melnechuck T. New York, Raven Press, 1980, pp 107–125

Ingvar DH, Franzen G: Distribution of cerebral activity in chronic schizophrenia. Lancet 2:1484–1486, 1974

Ingvar DH, Philipson L: Distribution of cerebral blood flow in the dominant hemisphere during motor ideation and motor performance. Ann Neurol 2:230–237, 1977

Ingvar DH, Sjolund B, Ardo A: Correlation between dominant EEG frequency, cerebral oxygen uptake and blood flow. Electroencephalogr Clin Neurophysiol 41:268–276, 1976

James AE Jr, Price RR, Rollo FD, et al: Nuclear magnetic resonance imaging: a promising technique. JAMA 247:1331–1334, 1982

Kety SS, Woodford RB, Harmel MH, et al: Cerebral blood flow and metabolism in schizophrenia. Am J Psychiatry 104:765–770, 1948

Kuhl DE, Barrio JR, Huang SC, et al: Quantifying local cerebral blood flow by N-Isopropyl-p-(^{123}) Iodoamphetamine (IMP) tomography. J Nucl Med 23:196–203, 1982

Lassen NA, Henriksen L, Holm S, et al: Cerebral blood flow tomography: xenon-133 compared with isopropyl-amphetamine-iodine-12: concise communication. J Nucl Med 24:17–21, 1983

Mathew RJ, Meyer JS, Francis DJ, et al: Cerebral blood flow in depression. Am J Psychiatry 137:1449–1450, 1980

Mathew RJ, Meyer JS, Francis DJ, et al: Regional cerebral blood flow in schizophrenia: a preliminary report. Am J Psychiatry 138:112–113, 1981

Matsui T, Hirano A: An atlas of the human brain for computerized tomography. Tokyo, Igaku-Shoin, 1978

McCulloch J, Savaki HE, Sokoloff L: Distribution of effects of haloperidol on energy metabolism in the brain. Brain Res 243:81–90, 1982

Morihisa JM, Duffy FH, Wyatt RJ: Topographic analysis of computer processed electroencephalography in schizophrenia, in Biological Markers in Psychiatry and Neurology. Edited by Usdin E, Hanin I. New York, Pergamon Press, 1982, pp 495–504

Morihisa JM, Duffy FH, Wyatt, RJ: Brain electrical activity mapping (BEAM) in schizophrenic patients. Arch Gen Psychiatry 40:719–728, 1983

Phelps ME, Juhl DE, Mazziotta JC: Metabolic mapping of the brain's response to visual stimulation: studies in humans. Science 211:1445–1448, 1981a

Phelps ME, Mazziotta JC, Kuhl DE, et al: Tomographic mapping of human cerebral metabolism: visual stimulation and deprivation. Neurology 31:517–529, 1981b

Phelps ME, Mazziotta JC, Huang SC: Study of cerebral function with positron computed tomography. J Cereb Blood Flow Metab 2:113–162, 1982

Risberg J: Regional cerebral blood flow measurement by ^{133}Xe-inhalation: methodology and applications in neuropsychology and psychiatry. Brain Lang 9:9–34, 1980

Rosenthal D: The Genain Quadruplets. New York, Basic Books, 1963

Rush AJ, Schlesser MA, Stokely E, et al: Cerebral blood flow in depression and mania, in Brain Imaging in Psychiatry and Neurology: Positron Emission Tomography and Other Techniques. Edited by Buchsbaum MS, Usdin E, Bunney WE Jr, et al. Pacific Grove, CA, Boxwood Press (in press)

Silfverskiold P, Gustafson L, Johansson BA, et al: RCBF in affective disorders, in Brain Imaging in Psychiatry and Neurology: Positron Emission Tomography and Other Techniques. Edited by Buchsbaum MS, Usdin E, Bunney WE Jr, et al. Pacific Grove, CA, Boxwood Press (in press)

Sokoloff L: Relationships among local functional activity, energy metabolism and blood flow in the central nervous system. Fed Proc 40:2311–2316, 1981

Sokoloff L: The radioactive deoxyglucose method, in Advances in Neurochemistry 4. Edited by Agranoff BW, Aprison MH. New York, Plenum, 1982, pp 1–81

Tolonen U, Sulg IA: Comparison of quantitative EEG parameters from four different analysis techniques in evaluation of relationships between EEG and CBF in brain infarction. Electroencephalogr Clin Neurophysiol 51:177–185, 1981

Wagner HN Jr, Burns HD, Dannals RF, et al: Imaging dopamine receptors in the human brain by positron tomography. Science 221:1264–1266, 1983

2

Regional Cerebral Blood Flow (rCBF) in Psychiatry: Methodological Issues

Isak Prohovnik, Ph.D.

2

Regional Cerebral Blood Flow (rCBF) in Psychiatry: Methodological Issues

Traditionally, measurements of regional cerebral blood flow (rCBF) have been confined to neurology and nuclear medicine. Only one laboratory had concentrated on using this technique in psychiatric studies (Risberg 1980). Recently, however, rCBF has been increasingly used in psychiatry (Mathew et al. 1982; Ariel et al. 1983; Uytdenhoef et al. 1983), and it seems appropriate at this time to examine the value and limitations of this method. The present article reviews selected methodological issues that may complicate the performance and interpretation of rCBF studies, with the aim of providing some means to evaluate published work and to plan further psychiatric research. In this paper, the term rCBF refers only to the two-dimensional, noninvasive methods that rely on inhalation or intravenous injection of xenon-133.

The growing interest of rCBF to psychiatry stems mostly from the fact that this technique can indirectly map cerebral metabolism and, by inference, neural activity or information processing. Regional metabolism and blood flow are closely coupled in the human brain in the absence of gross pathology, and since psychiatric patients rarely present acute neurological abnormalities that might disrupt this coupling, one may infer regional metabolism from flow.

THEORY OF rCBF

The theoretical work leading to present rCBF technology began with that of Kety, Zierler and others. For an excellent review of the theory of tracer kinetics, see Lassen and Perl (1979). In brief, the parameter most directly measured by tracer kinetics is mean transit time (MTT): a small quantity of a tracer is introduced into the blood stream, and its quantity is measured in a region of interest as a function of time. MTT is simply the observed average time in which the tracer molecules traverse the region of interest. Given an appropriate tracer, this value is assumed to be identical to the MTT of blood itself. Flow is computed from MTT by the following equation:

$$F = V/T \tag{1}$$

where F is blood flow (ml/min), V is the distribution volume of the tracer (ml), and T is MTT (min).

In applying this simple formula to physiological measurements in vivo, the V term is difficult to define: not only is the cerebral blood volume of man imprecisely known, but it also varies widely in some situations, by as much as 100 percent. Quantitative estimates of flow cannot, therefore, be achieved by nondiffusible tracers, such as those used in angiography. To solve this problem, tracers that freely diffuse across the blood-brain barrier, such as N_2O or xenon, are employed; these equilibrate rapidly between blood and brain parenchyma, and therefore their distribution volume is equivalent to tissue volume (since cerebral blood volume is negligible in comparison). The concentration of tracer in tissue will then be a function of its blood concentration and the partition coefficient λ. Dividing both sides of equation 1 by an arbitrary tissue weight, e.g., 100 g, yields:

$$F/W = V/WT \tag{2}$$

and now f (relative flow, in ml/100 g/min) can be substituted for F/W, λ for V/W, and k (the decay constant, in min^{-1}) for $1/T$:

$$f = k\lambda \tag{3}$$

Thus, given k (which is directly measurable from the observed tracer concentrations in tissue and arterial blood) and λ (which is usually assumed), flow can be computed. Note, however, that a measure of absolute flow through the tissue is no longer obtained, but only one of relative flow. If significant atrophy is present, it will not be detected by observed flow values, which reflect activity in the remaining functional tissue (but see discussion in later sections). Additionally, we assume λ to be normal in psychiatric patients, although it is known to vary in neoplasms and possibly in other pathological conditions.

The mathematical procedures for deriving k from observed clearance curves are beyond the scope of this paper; they have been described by Obrist et al. (1975) and Prohovnik et al. (1983).

METHODOLOGY: PHYSICAL ASPECTS

In order to perform rCBF measurements, tracer concentrations must be monitored in the region of interest throughout the measurement period, usually 10 to 15 minutes. This is done by scintillation detectors aimed at the regions from outside the skull. Tracer is administered by 1-min inhalation or intravenous injection. Each detector records a "clearance curve" of the arrival and gradual elimination of tracer from the relevant region. Analysis is performed by matching a theoretical function, determined by the physiological model, to the observed values.

Count Rate

One of the major determinants of the quality of data analysis is the count rate observed. Radioactivity counts are described by Poisson distribution, where variance is equal to the mean. Most current methods gather samples every five or six seconds, for a sample count rate of 1,000 to 5,000. Those count rates are obtained at the peak of the curve, usually occurring one to two minutes after tracer administration. At the start and end of measurement counts may be as low as 200 to 300. Using the low radiation doses necessary to perform many repeated measurements on normal volunteers, and using short measurement times for similar reasons, some studies may yield unreliable data because of low counts. One way of improving such measures without increasing radiation exposure is to monitor a larger "energy window," that is to include low-energy counts in the calculations. Using wider energy windows certainly increases count rates, but it may also reduce spatial resolution and increase sensitivity to artifacts.

Goodness of Fit

The analysis of clearance curves is performed by fitting a theoretical function to the observed values. The fit, however, is never completely right or wrong, and the solution not always appropriate. Most commercial programs supply some information about goodness of fit to indicate when a solution is less than optimal, usually because of noisy data. This information is seldom exhaustive or definitive, and the operator must perform further tests to determine the source and severity of the problem. Risberg and Prohovnik (1981) provide a detailed discussion of this issue. It should be emphasized here, however, that automatically accepting all computer solutions is sometimes imprudent.

Temporal Resolution

Flow values reflect a weighted average of cerebral activity during the monitoring period. Tracer washout is usually monitored for 10 minutes following administration, rarely up to 15 minutes. Simpler models, which allow less rigorous quantification, make it possible to perform measurements in about 4 minutes. The more complex compartmental models, however, deteriorate rapidly when measurement times are shortened below 10 minutes. Some flow indices, such as the initial slope index (ISI), are less affected by short measurements than are the primary parameters (Risberg et al. 1975). Using longer monitoring periods, better estimates can be obtained of white matter and extracranial tissue flows (Obrist et al. 1967), but a significantly longer measurement period would limit the clinical utility of the method and it is not currently used.

Temporal resolution also determines the sampling time and the ability to perform repeated measurement rapidly. As earlier mentioned, the standard sampling period is 5 to 6 seconds. Attempts have been made to shorten it (Nilsson et al. 1982); rapid sampling, if achieved without significant degradation of statistical counting reliability, may allow extraction of more precise information from the clearance curves. Since xenon has a higher affinity for adipose tissue, and therefore remains bound there longer than in the brain, it had been assumed that rCBF measurements cannot be repeated more frequently than at intervals of about one hour. Risberg (1980) introduced a simple and effective correction for this remaining activity, and now it is possible to repeat measurements immediately.

Spatial Resolution

rCBF systems are currently available with up to 16 detectors for each hemisphere. The collimators usually have an internal diameter of 15 to 20 mm and are about 20 mm long. Optical resolution at about 10 mm from the collimator surface is about 20 to 40 mm (see, for example, Stump and Williams 1980). Because of Compton scatter and the attenuation of xenon-133 energy in tissue, true resolution is probably somewhat worse, but rigorous studies have not been performed.

A special problem for resolution is "crosstalk," which is the contamination of a detector by radiation originating in the contralateral hemisphere. Bolmsjo (1981) and Hartmann and Kummer (1983) recently studied this problem and concluded that 5 to 30 percent of observed counts originate in the contralateral hemisphere. These figures are representative of the literature; the exact figures corresponding to particular applications depend on geometrical considerations, collimation, the energy window employed, and other factors. Crosstalk reduces the sensitivity of rCBF to flow assymmetries; detected asymmetries may be assumed to be underestimated.

Because of the importance of repeated studies and the use of controls in rCBF, attention should also be given to the reliability of detector positioning, that is to ensuring that each detector is placed in the same position for each measurement. Some systems are now equipped with positioning aids, and Farrar (1981) has described another method for this purpose. Data obtained without careful attention to the reliability of positioning will be noisy and will display reduced spatial resolution.

METHODOLOGY: PHYSIOLOGICAL ASPECTS

Since the analysis procedure consists of fitting a theoretical model to observed data, the nature and validity of the model play a major role in determining the quality of results. Two central aspects to consider in rCBF modeling are artifacts (defined here as any information unrelated to cerebral blood flow) and compartmentalization (gray versus white matter). There are additional considerations in interpreting the significance of data (normal variation, vascular and metabolic effects, and sensitivity to different conditions).

Artifacts

The two artifacts that generated most concern in the early use of noninvasive rCBF were related to recirculation and extracranial tissue influence. Both have since been addressed successfully (Obrist et al. 1975). Concern about one artifact remained, however, an artifact reflecting direct and indirect counts from xenon in respiratory air (air-passage artifact APA). This artifact could not be separated by the proposed analysis, and therefore the curve-fitting procedure began only when xenon concentrations dropped markedly in respiratory air. Since then, there have been several attempts to eliminate this artifact and allow a "full-curve analysis" (e.g., Jablonski et al. 1979; Hazelrig et al. 1981; Nilsson et al. 1982). The model containing this artifact was recently found to be inadequate (Risberg and Prohovnik 1981), and a more comprehensive model was developed (Prohovnik et al. 1981). The last model assumes an additional artifact arising from xenon in arterial blood. This model and associated changes in algorithms were extensively tested by computer simulations and found to perform satisfactorily (Prohovnik et al. 1983). Verification in man is still incomplete, however, and the magnitude of errors generated by different models in vivo is not yet known.

Compartmentalization

Current views ascribe the rCBF signal to two cerebral flow compartments, fast and slow. The fast compartment is taken to correspond to gray matter, and the slow compartment to white matter, contaminated by slow flow in scalp tissues. The values obtained for both compartments in normal brains are in good agreement with expected values, but difficulties usually arise in the presence of data degradation. Under such conditions, the algorithms cannot accurately separate the two compartments and a so-called "slippage" occurs. The usual form of this slippage is an overestimation of both fast and slow compartment clearance and a diminution of the relative size of the fast compartment. The primary flow parameters are then inadequate to characterize true perfusion. Under these conditions, it is better to use flow indices that reflect mean tissue perfusion with some variable degree of preference to gray or white matter. This solution has been proposed by Risberg et al. (1975), using the ISI parameter, and Obrist and Wilkinson (1980), using the CBF15 parameter.

Confounding Variables

As in taking any physiological measurement, systemic factors should be controlled in using rCBF. Two examples relevant to psychiatric studies are arterial CO_2 tension and hemoglobin values. Carbon dioxide is a potent vasodilator, and cerebral blood flow (CBF) is highly sensitive to its acute changes. A patient who is anxious during the measurement may hyperventilate and thereby reduce $PaCO_2$. CBF will decrease accordingly. This flow reduction does not reflect reduced cerebral metabolism and should be corrected if the investigator is seeking values that reflect cortical activity. Anorexic patients may often be anemic, with low hemoglobin values. Due to the affinity of xenon for hemoglobin, the blood-brain partition coefficient should be adjusted in such cases to achieve a valid correlation between blood flow and metabolism. (The correlation may be compromised additionally by associated changes in blood viscosity and oxygen capacity.) The interpretation of rCBF is more difficult when subjects have neurological abnormalities, such as ischemia, when the coupling between rCBF and cerebral metabolism may be variable, but considering such cases is beyond the scope of this article.

Medication may also confound rCBF findings. Low or abnormal rCBF in a patient may result from the metabolic effects of medication (haldol, for example, Nilsson et al. 1977) or from the changes it may effect in cerebrovascular control mechanisms (as in the case of lithium and amitriptyline, for example, Preskorn et al. 1981), or from both.

Data Significance

A multitude of secondary parameters can be computed from rCBF models. Primary parameters range from two to six, but more than twenty secondary parameters have been proposed (Stump and Williams 1980). The secondary parameters may be more reliable in the presence of noise, as the previous section indicated. On the other hand, they vary widely in sensitivity, and the physiology underlying some of them is unclear (although all have rigorously defined mathematical meaning).

Again, indices vary in sensitivity, reliability, and normal variation (Risberg and Prohovnik 1981). Reliability and sensitivity are usually negatively correlated. In addition, different indices may suggest opposing trends, because of noise in the data or problems of compartmentalization. This is usually not a severe constraint in analyzing group data, but may distort the analysis of individual cases. Figure 1 illustrates the problem with a clinical case of a 44-year-old male chronic schizophrenic (who had negative CT and EEG results). When the first rCBF measurement was performed, the patient was catatonic. The results show normal average flow for three parameters (f_1, ISI, and CBF15), but an abnormal regional pattern that is most obvious in f_1. Regional flow patterns in all three parameters are very similar. A second measurement was performed after intravenous injection of diazepam (3.5 mg). The patient then dramatically improved, talking, walking, and requesting lunch. Compared to measures taken when the subject was unmedicated, $PeCO_2$ was unchanged, mean arterial blood pressure (MABP) was slightly reduced, and CBF was much lower. His flows, however, differ among the three parameters: f_1 and ISI

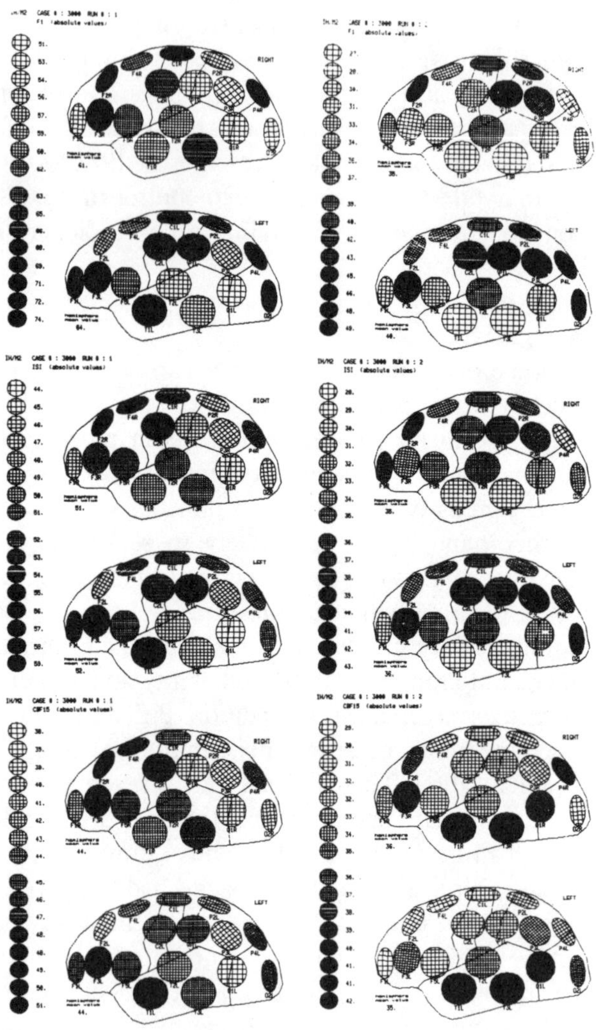

Figure 1. The results of rCBF for a 44-year-old man with chronic schizophrenia who was in a catatonic state (run 1, left column) and when improved after diazepam (run 2, right column). Flow is estimated using three parameters: f_1 (upper rows), ISI (middle rows) and CBF15 (lower rows). The right hemisphere is always presented above the left, and mean hemispheric values are noted at the lower left corner of each hemisphere. Regional values are depicted by a gray scale, different for each condition and parameter, provided at the left side of each pair of hemispheres.

show parietal flows higher than temporal, whereas CBF15 demonstrates the opposite. ISI and CBF15 reveal no hemispheric asymmetry, whereas f_1 indicates the right hemisphere flow to be lower than the left. This case is unusually difficult to interpret, but less extreme examples are not rare. In this case, discrepancies were caused by movement artifacts, xenon leaks, and very low values of CBF, which lead to problems in compartmentalization. Interpretation based on a single parameter without careful examination of clearance curves would probably lead to erroneous conclusions. Until a better understanding of the indices is achieved, it is prudent to examine at least three: a sensitive one (for example, f_1), a reliable one (for example, CBF15), and the relative compartment weights. Such practice also helps reduce the disadvantage of measuring relative flow: some indices, especially those that reflect compartment size more than clearance, may be more sensitive to the reduced volume of viable tissue that may occur in ischemia or atrophy, conditions that may be relevant to dementia research.

Serious problems emerge in statistically evaluating rCBF data, in view of the preceding: one may be faced with 10 parameters derived from 32 detectors for each measurement occasion in each subject. There are complex and variable relations among the parameters and detectors, and it is not yet clear how to evaluate the significance of any effect. Statistical analysis of rCBF data remains a major challenge for research (Wood 1980).

In addition, absolute rCBF values are normally quite variable, possibly because of the sensitivity of the technique to transient psychophysiological states. The normal baseline ("resting") measurement yields a wide range of values, which may be related to demographic variables, such as age and sex, or to the influence of uncontrolled subjective states. Relative flow patterns are more stable, and symmetry is normally preserved. Nonetheless, "resting" baseline rCBF values are of questionable diagnostic utility in psychiatry. This has led recently to the use of "activation" rCBF measurements, in which a subject is monitored while performing a task. Activation rCBF measurements are becoming common and show definite potential. Their interpretation may be complicated, however, by the assumption that a particular task is perceived and performed in the same way by different patients and controls. It is advisable, when using such measures, to document the comparable performance of experimental groups.

SUMMARY AND COMMENTS

The present review has briefly introduced some methodological issues for rCBF as it is applied in psychiatry. This information should help the reader to evaluate published results and plan further research. Because of limitation of space, rCBF instrumentation and procedures are not described here, and the methodological issues are only mentioned rather than analyzed in detail. The interested reader can find more exhaustive treatments in the literature cited.

Despite the complexities reviewed here, there is overwhelming evidence of the validity and reliability of the rCBF method. Many of its methodological problems can be circumvented by repeated studies within patients, with appropriate attention to effective experimental controls. A major potential of the rCBF method may lie in correlating its results with clinical status, treatment variables, and diagnostic subtypes. The patient whose record is shown in Figure 1 did demonstrate a dramatic change of behavior after being administered diazepam, and though there were discrepancies among the different parameters of flow, his CBF was clearly reduced by the medication, indicating a possible disinhibitory effect. As the present volume indicates, much information can be gleaned in rCBF studies of the "activated" brain, that is, during subjects' performance of behavioral tasks. The next few years should provide exciting tests of the theoretical and clinical contributions of rCBF in psychiatry.

References

Ariel RN, Golden CJ, Berg RA, et al: Regional cerebral blood flow in schizophrenics. Arch Gen Psychiatry 40:258–263, 1983

Bolmsjo M: Hemisphere cross-talk and signal overlapping in bilateral rCBF measurements using ^{133}Xe, in The Physical and Physiological Aspects of Xenon Isotopes in Nuclear Medical Applications. Unpublished doctoral dissertation, Department of Radiation Physics, Lund University, 1981

Farrar JK: A computerized technique for the display and comparison of regional cerebral blood flow data. Stroke 12:22–26, 1981

Hartmann A, Kummer RV: Atraumatic measurement of regional cerebral blood flow: methods and reliability tests. Fortschr Neurol Psychiatr 1983 (in press)

Hazelrig JB, Katholi CR, Blauenstein UW, et al: Total curve analysis of regional cerebral blood flow with ^{133}Xe inhalation. IEEE Trans Biomed Eng 28:603–616, 1981

Jablonski T, Prohovnik I, Risberg J, et al: Fourier analysis of ^{133}Xe inhalation curves. Acta Neurol Scand 60 (Suppl 72):216–217, 1979

Lassen NA, Perl W: Tracer Kinetic Methods in Medical Physiology. New York, Raven Press, 1979

Mathew RJ, Duncan GC, Weiman ML, et al: Regional cerebral blood flow in schizophrenia. Arch Gen Psychiatry 39:1121–1124, 1982

Nilsson A, Risberg J, Johanson M, et al: Regional changes of cerebral blood flow during haloperidol therapy in patients with paranoid symptoms. Acta Neurol Scand 56 (Suppl 64):478–479, 1977

Nilsson BG, Ryding E, Ingvar DH: Quantitative airway artifact compensation at regional cerebral blood flow measurements with radioactive gases. J Cereb Blood Flow Metab 2:73–78, 1982

Obrist WD, Wilkinson WE: The noninvasive Xe-133 method: evaluation of CBF indices, in Cerebral Circulation. Edited by Bes A, Geraud G. Amsterdam, Excerpta Medica, 1980.

Obrist WD, Thompson HK, King HC, et al: Determination of regional cerebral blood flow by inhalation of [133]xenon. Circ Res 20:124–135, 1967

Obrist WD, Thompson HK, Wang HS, et al: Regional cerebral blood flow estimated by [133]xenon inhalation. Stroke 6:245–256, 1975

Preskorn SH, Irwin GH, Simpson S, et al: Medical therapies for mood disorders alter the blood-brain barrier. Science 213:469–471, 1981

Prohovnik I, Risberg J, Mubrin Z, et al: Further improvements of the ^{133}Xe inhalation method. J Cereb Blood Flow Metab 1 (Suppl. 1): 108–109, 1981

Prohovnik I, Knudsen E, Risberg J: Accuracy of models and algorithms for determination of fast-compartment flow by noninvasive ^{133}Xe clearance, in Functional Radionuclide Imaging of the Brain. Edited by Magistretti PL. New York, Raven Press, 1983

Risberg J: Regional cerebral blood flow measurements by ^{133}Xe inhalation: methodology and applications in neuropsychology and psychiatry. Brain Lang 9:9–34, 1980

Risberg J, Prohovnik I: rCBF Measurements by ^{133}Xe inhalation: recent methodological advances, in Progress in Nuclear Medicine, Volume 7. Edited by Juge O, Donath A. Karger, Basel, 1981, pp 70–81

Risberg J, Ali Z, Wilson EM, et al: Regional cerebral blood flow by [133]xenon inhalation: preliminary evaluation of an initial slope index in patients with unstable flow compartments. Stroke 6:511–524, 1975

Stump DA, Williams R: The noninvasive measurement of regional cerebral circulation. Brain Lang 9:35–46, 1980

Uytdenhoef P, Portelange P, Jacquy J, et al: Regional cerebral blood flow and lateralized hemispheric dysfunction in depression. Br J Psychiatry 143:128–132, 1983

Wood F: Theoretical, methodological and statistical implications of the inhalation rCBF technique for the study of brain-behavior relationships. Brain Lang 9:1–8, 1980

3

Regional Cerebral Blood Flow in Psychiatry: Application to Clinical Research

Karen Faith Berman, M.D.
Daniel R. Weinberger, M.D.
John M. Morihisa, M.D.
Ronald F. Zec, Ph.D.

3

Regional Cerebral Blood Flow in Psychiatry: Application to Clinical Research

New techniques of "brain imaging" have recently captured the interest of the psychiatric community. This is not surprising in view of their potential to localize and to physiologically characterize mental phenomena in the living human brain. Prior to the advent of such innovative techniques, we could only speculate about the origin of these phenomena. For example, the hallucinations of a schizophrenic that are phenomenologically similar to those of someone with a limbic seizure disorder might also be of limbic origin. Brain-imaging technology might confirm this if it identified the physiological correlates (for example, changes in cerebral metabolism) of such mental phenomena.

The characteristics of an ideal brain-imaging system for psychiatric research include the following: (1) noninvasiveness so as not to contaminate the physiological "landscape" by creating extraneous cognitive sets; (2) sufficient spatial resolution to measure important structures like the limbic system and basal ganglia; (3) sufficient temporal resolution to study transient mental phenomena; (4) applicability to the study of psychiatric patients, who might resist motor restraints or other procedural inconveniences. Unfortunately, present method fulfills all these criteria. Those methods with better spatial resolution tend to be more physically restrictive or invasive, and those that are less invasive have poorer spatial resolution.

Of the techniques now used for functional brain imaging, the measure of regional cerebral blood flow (rCBF) by inhalation of xenon-133 has unique advantages in psychiatric studies of higher cortical function. Xenon-133 gas is a low-energy gamma-ray-emitting radioisotope that is inhaled by the subject and used to trace regional cerebral blood flow, a parameter closely related to cortical glucose metabolism. Since xenon is freely diffusible and inert, it exchanges readily between blood and tissue, yet fails to affect metabolic processes. If a tissue is first saturated with xenon-133 and then allowed to desaturate, its radioactivity diminishes as a direct function of the blood flow to the area. Since gamma rays penetrate brain tissue and skull, external monitoring of this change is possible. Monitoring the desaturation of contiguous cortical regions provides a regional map of blood flow and, by inference, of cortical metabolism.

In deciding to employ xenon-133 rCBF in psychiatric research, it is important to consider the relative merits and limitations of the technique. The method is noninvasive, quick, and relatively easy to carry out. Because it exposes the subject to little radiation, a number of studies can be performed on the same individual in fairly rapid succession. The technique thus allows various cognitive or psychological "activation" studies in addition to "resting" studies. It is also possible to study changing clinical states and medication conditions with a subject serving as his or her own control. Another major advantage of the technique is its relatively short temporal resolution of less than 10 minutes. This allows the study of blood flow and, by inference, metabolic concomitants of transient mental states. The hardware for xenon-133 rCBF is relatively inexpensive (equipment and installation are less than $140,000); the isotope is readily available and remarkably cheap; and, unlike the radionuclides used in positron emission tomography (PET), xenon-133 does not require a cyclotron for its production. The cost of xenon-133 per study is approximately $15.

Compared to more sophisticated techniques, however, the

method has important limitations. It has limited spatial resolution compared to PET scanning (an estimated 2 to 4 cm of cortical surface for rCBF compared to less than 1 cm for current PET scanners). Unlike tomographic techniques that can image deep subcortical structures, xenon-133 rCBF yields only a two-dimensional topography of superficial cortical metabolism. Certain problems like "cross-talk" are intrinsic to this method (see Chapter 2), and limit its sensitivity to regional differences and hemispheric asymmetries.

In the following sections we describe aspects of the xenon-133 inhalation technique as it has been modified in our lab, as well as a number of considerations and prerequisites for setting up such a facility. We also discuss the processes by which we technically and clinically validated the methods used. Several case studies follow along with descriptions of the approaches we are taking in investigating psychiatric illnesses with rCBF. Since the concept of a relation between brain functional activity, metabolism, and blood flow has a long history, both in theory and in practice, we first briefly review some of this history and some of the principles involved.

BACKGROUND

In 1890 Charles Roy and Charles Sherrington observed that seconds after the onset of an epileptic seizure a swelling of the brain occurred, suggesting an increase in its supply of blood. About 25 years later, Joseph Bancroft elaborated on the idea that blood flow to a tissue varies with its functional activity and metabolism. He hypothesized that enhanced functional activity can be sustained only by increasing the rate of oxygen consumption, and thus the flow of oxygenated blood, to the tissue. In 1937 Carl Schmidt and James Hendrix recorded a strictly localized increase in blood flow to the visual cortex when they shined a small spot of light on the retina of a cat.

In 1944 Seymour Kety and Carl Schmidt developed the nitrous oxide technique to determine whole brain mean blood flow in humans. The method specified a 10-minute inhalation of 15 percent nitrous oxide and the sampling of venous and arterial blood to observe the rate at which the brain was saturated and desaturated with this gas. Application of the Fick principle yielded a measure of mean cerebral blood flow (Kety and Schmidt 1945).

In the early 1960s Ingvar and others measured regional cortical blood flow by injecting xenon-133 into the carotid artery. They externally monitored the arrival and elimination of radioactivity in cortical areas supplied by carotid circulation using a gamma camera (Ingvar et al. 1965). Since gamma rays from deep structures were known to be markedly attenuated, researchers assumed that radioactivity monitored in this way was primarily that of the superficial cerebral cortex.

Mallett and Veall later introduced a noninvasive technique to measure regional cerebral blood flow using the inhalation of xenon-133 gas. Their procedure specified 5 minutes of inhalation and external monitoring of the elimination of radioactivity over 20 minutes (Mallett and Veall 1965; Veall and Mallett 1966).

In the early 1970s Walter Obrist designed a two-compartment mathematical model to interpret desaturation curves. The model analyzes cerebral flow in terms of a fast-clearing (gray matter) compartment and a slow-clearing (white matter) compartment (Obrist et al. 1971; Obrist et al. 1975). Obrist's mathematical model made the technique practical and attractive.

Preliminary studies of rCBF in psychiatric patients have been inconclusive and sometimes contradictory. In 1948, Kety found no difference in mean cerebral blood flow (CBF) between a group of control subjects and a group of schizophrenic patients using the nitrous oxide technique (Kety et al. 1948). Using the xenon-133 intracarotid technique, however, David Ingvar conducted a series of studies in the 1970s from which there emerged an intriguing finding: while normal subjects at rest showed relatively greater blood flow to frontal than to posterior cortex—the so-called "normal hyperfrontal pattern"—chronic schizophrenics, despite showing normal mean CBF, showed relatively reduced flow in frontal compared to posterior brain regions. Although potentially important, this work suffered a number of methodological limitations, including failure to control for medication state and subject age, in addition to problems inherent in the invasiveness of the procedure. Careful replication and extension of these findings certainly seemed warranted.

Using the noninvasive inhalation technique Matthew and his colleagues (1982) reported decreased mean blood flow in schizophrenics, but no regional differences. This study focused only on the resting state, however, and since it is unlikely that the experience of sitting with the eyes closed at rest is the same for one individual at two sittings, much less for different individuals (see, for example, Mazziotta et al. 1982), the interpretation of such data is inherently problematic.

We felt there remained many unresolved questions that could be addressed by well-designed rCBF studies. Our efforts to develop a research strategy and the problems we confronted in doing so are detailed in the following section.

TECHNICAL CONSIDERATIONS

Radiation Safety

The use of radionuclides requires familiarity with issues of radiation safety and the requirements of the Nuclear Regulatory Commission (NRC) in addition to the usual concerns about the safety of patients and research subjects. It should be emphasized that the risks and problems of using xenon-133 gas, a low-energy gamma-ray emitter, are minimal compared with those encountered in using positron emitters or some substances common in biochemistry labs like iodine-125, phosporous-32, carbon-14, and tritium. Nonetheless, procedures and provisions for monitoring the environment and personnel exposure are still necessary when using xenon-133, as is extensive documentation. Nuclear Regulatory Commission guidelines limit radiation exposure for research subjects and workers to 5,000 mrads per year (1,250 per quarter) to the whole body, active blood-forming organs, or gonads. National Institutes of Health (NIH) regulations further limit volunteers for research to exposure of 3,000 mrad per year to any single tissue. Exposure resulting from a single rCBF procedure has been estimated at less than 5 mrad to the bone marrow (whole body) and at less than 200 mrad to the lung (Deshmukh and Meyer 1978; Obrist, personal communication).

The use of a radioactive gas poses special problems in that adequate ventilation of the laboratory is mandatory. For each radioisotope, the NRC specifies a maximum permissible concentration (MPC), that is, the maximum activity of a radioactive gas permitted within a given volume of air or water. MPC values are expressed as microcuries (μCi) per ml. The MPC for xenon-133 in the laboratory is 1×10^{-5} μCi/ml for a period of 40 hours (40 "MPC hours") in any consecutive 7 days (Code of Federal Regulations Title 10, Part 20, Section 103, and Part 20, Appendix B, Table 1). In our laboratory, this required installation of an extensive exhaust system to achieve air flow greater than 500 cubic feet per minute. Ventilation is checked regularly with a flowmeter, and room air is continuously monitored with a XenoGard® model 36-751 (Victoreen, Inc.), which provides a cumulative record of MPC hours. Sufficient air exchange, adequate personnel training, appropriate emergency plans, and waste disposal must all be fully documented in applying for the NRC license to handle radioactive xenon. In some settings, collaborating with a department of nuclear medicine would eliminate the need to implement these steps de novo.

Description of the System

A commercially available gas delivery system (Radx Ventl-Con II®) is used to determine and adjust the concentration of xenon-133 and to deliver the gas precisely and accurately to the subject. This delivery system required considerable additional lead shielding for safe operation. We have found that using a snorkle-like mouthpiece together with a cushioned nose clip results in less gas leakage and data of better quality. The mouthpiece is also less intimidating to most subjects than the more widely used face mask.

Blood flow is determined with a 32-probe dynamic rCBF analysis system designed by the Harshaw Chemical and Electronics Company. The 32 extracranial scintillation detectors are arranged radially over both hemispheres in 16 homologous, right-left pairs (Figure 1). Each consists of thallium-activated sodium

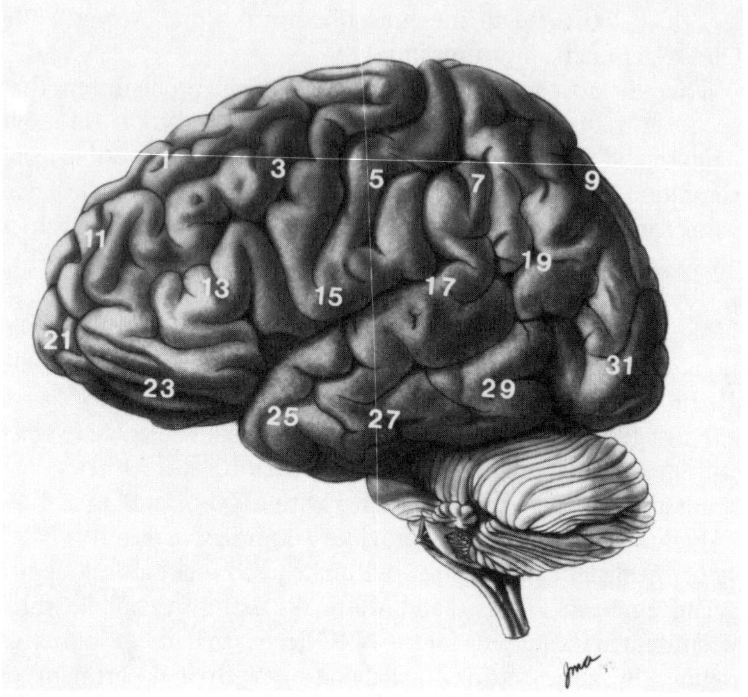

Figure 1. Approximate locations of the 16 left hemisphere probes with respect to the cerebral cortex.

iodide, NaI(Tl), crystal, ½ in. in diameter and ¾ in. long, attached to a collimator 25 mm long and 4 mm thick. The collimator is a lead cylinder used to maximize the probability that each crystal monitors only photons from a discrete, "focused" area. Each NaI(Tl) scintillation crystal converts the energy of photons into visible light (scintillation counts). It transmits "counts" to a photomultiplier tube (PMT) that converts the light scintillations into an electrical signal for computer processing. Counts from the head probes are sampled in 6-sec epochs. A sample of the expired air is simultaneously monitored for end-tidal carbon dioxide concentration ($PeCO_2$) with a Capnograph (Beckman LB-3) and for radioactivity concentration by a separate sodium iodide detector, or "air probe," which collects radiation counts every 0.6 sec. Since expiratory end-tidal xenon-133 counts (the "air curve") yield very close estimates of actual arterial concentrations (Veall and Mallett 1966), these concentrations can be used to correct for the small amount of xenon-133 that recirculates. This eliminates the need for invasive arterial monitoring. The data from each of the 32 head probes is used to generate a clearance curve that reflects the arrival and gradual elimination of radioactivity from the relevant cortical region.

In contrast to the practice in most rCBF labs, we presented visual stimuli with the subject seated rather than reclining and modified a dental chair for this purpose. This arrangement proved to have an important advantage over having subjects be recumbent. With the subject seated, external landmarks (the orbitomeatal line and the positions of the frontopolar leads of the standard international 10-20 electroencephalograph system) are located and used to ensure consistent alignment of the 32 external detectors.

An entire study takes approximately 16 min. After the probes are carefully positioned, the room lights are dimmed. While the subject breathes room air, we measure "background radiation" for 4 min to control for any radioactivity that may be present in the subject or the environment. For resting procedures the subject sits without moving and with eyes closed. If an activation procedure is to be carried out, it is begun after the third minute of background counting (1 min before inhalation of xenon-133 begins) and is continued throughout the session. After the 4 min background count the subject breathes a mixture of room air and xenon-133 at a concentration of 5 to 7 mCi/l for 1 min and then room air for the next 11 min. Using a mouthpiece with the nose clamped, the subject does not know when xenon inhalation begins or ends. The entire 16 min of 6-sec radiation counts (the clearance curve) from each of the 32 extracranial detectors and the air probe are stored on a floppy disc and analyzed. These "raw data" can also be displayed on a graphics terminal. Printout of continuous $PeCO_2$ is simultaneously available. $PeCO_2$ is an important parameter because CBF varies directly with it.

We use software designed by Walter Obrist (Obrist et al. 1975) for data analysis. For each of the 32 clearance curves (raw data), the algorithm corrects for background and recirculating xenon-133 and performs a least-squares curve-fitting procedure to "tighten" the data and, with iterations, deconvolutes it according to the two-compartment model. Two overlapping desaturation curves result, a fast-clearing or gray matter compartment with a steep slope, and a slow-clearing or white matter compartment with a gradual slope. Various indices of gray matter, white matter, and whole tissue blood flow as well as relative tissue compartment weights can be mathematically derived from these curves. These have been discussed in detail elsewhere (Obrist et al. 1975; Obrist and Wilkinson 1980; Risberg et al. 1975). Peak counts and "goodness of fit" to the mathematical model can also be examined.

In our blood flow studies we measure a number of physiological indices simultaneously, including pulse rate, $PeCO_2$, respiratory rate, and galvanic skin response. We allow at least 30 minutes between each procedure.

REFINING THE METHOD: rCBF AS ASSAY

It is important to emphasize that, despite the relative ease with which a blood flow study can be carried out, it cannot be considered a simple "black box" system for which validity can be assumed. On the contrary, as in any assay, many factors can adversely affect the quality of the data. Those variables that can be controlled should be, and those that cannot be controlled should be fully understood, minimized, and taken into account in evaluating the data. What are optimal substrate concentrations? What is the sensitivity of the assay and what affects its sensitivity? How reliable and reproducible are results? What are optimal conditions for the assay? The following discussion is by no means exhaustive, but provides examples of some of the factors we examined in order to minimize methodological artifacts.

Slippage and Other Hazards

Several methodological artifacts are inherent in rCBF. "Slippage," for example, is a quirk of the two-compartment model that occurs when the mathematical algorithm is unable to properly separate the fast and slow (or gray and white) compartments.

Slippage is assumed to have occurred when gray matter flow values for a right and left homologous probe pair differ by more than 10 percent and at the same time are inversely related to the relative tissue compartment weights for these probes. While from zero to ten pairs may show slippage in a given study, the reasons for this are not clear. We examined the following factors in attempting to control and define slippage:

Study Time.   We found that the longer the time period available for analysis, and the more data available for consideration, the fewer the number of slippages. "Start fit time" refers to the time that passes from the beginning of xenon inhalation (minute zero) to when curve-fitting and data analysis begin. To avoid distortions in the radiation counts of the head probes by high concentrations of xenon-133 in the airway passages, no data are included in the computations until expired air concentration decreases to 20 percent of its peak. The time at which this occurs (usually less than 3 minutes) marks the start fit time. Start fit times vary from study to study owing to a number of factors including subjects' breathing patterns. Since our current system can analyze up to 12 minutes of data, the actual time period analyzed in any particular study is equal to 12 minutes minus the start fit time for that study. Thus, the start fit time is inversely correlated with the time period analyzed. We examined start fit times and number of slippages for 245 consecutive studies and, as we expected, found a significant direct correlation between start fit time and number of slippages (Pearson $r = .25$, $p < .0002$). This correlation accounts for only 6.25 percent of the variance, however, and, as we will see, a number of other factors affect slippage.

Energy Window.   Energy filters are set to screen out radiation of higher or lower energy than that of the specific photon of interest (referred to as the "photopeak"). For xenon-133 the gamma ray photopeak is at 81 KeV. X-ray emission also occurs with the decay of xenon-133, and its photopeak is at 31 KeV. We examined 137 consecutive studies, 59 done with an energy "window" of 100 KeV (i.e., counting both photopeaks and, thus, increasing total counts) and 78 done with a window of 40 KeV (excluding the x-ray peak). Start fit times were significantly shorter (providing a longer period for analysis) in studies conducted with the narrower (40 KeV) window (2.25 min $\pm$ 0.3 versus 2.50 min $\pm$ 0.3, $p < .001$). Slippages were accordingly reduced from an average of 4.5 to 3.75 per study.

Count Rate.   The higher the count rate, the less subject are data to random variation, the better the counting statistics, and the fewer the slippages that occur.

Location.   It was important to discover whether slippages occurred randomly with regard to location or whether data from certain extracranial positions were more prone to this artifact. If found to be random, such spurious values could be assumed to not affect grouped or averaged data in any systematic way and need not be discarded. In examining over 300 studies we found no significant relation between slippage and the location of probes.

Taking all the factors above into account, we felt that we had minimized slippage and ensured that when it occurred it was random with respect to region recorded.

Reliability

As in any assay, we were obligated to determine the reproducibility and reliability of the data. We first studied 11 young (age 26.2 ± 5.2 years), healthy, normal volunteers at rest on two consecutive days at the same time of day. Table 1 shows resulting means for blood flow in gray matter (f1) in left and right hemisphere for each day and the differences in values from day 1 to day 2. There are no systematic differences in the values of repeated tests; the test-retest values are highly correlated. The standard deviations of the day-to-day differences were 5.23 for left hemisphere and 5.63 for right hemisphere, or approximately 7 percent of the respective means. Thus, day-to-day changes of more than 14 percent (two standard deviations) can be considered statistically significant at the 0.05 level. These 95-percent confidence limits are quite similar to those of Obrist et al. (1975) (14 per-

Table 1. Test-Retest Values for Gray Matter Cerebral Blood Flow in 11 Subjects

	Left Hemisphere		Right Hemisphere		
	Mean	SD	Mean	SD	PeCO$_2$
Day 1	78.55	8.98	79.25	8.26	47.4
Day 2	77.74	6.80	78.58	6.40	46.5
Mean Difference (Day 1 − Day 2)	0.81	5.23	0.67	5.63	...
Correlation Coefficient	0.815	...	0.734	...	...
95% Confidence Limits	...	13.4%	...	14.3%	...

NOTE. Figures express mean cerebral blood flow (f1) in ml/100 g/min. SD = standard deviation. PeCO$_2$ = end-tidal carbon dioxide concentration.

cent) using higher count rates and a technique of poorer spatial resolution. In fact, the reliability of our data is superior to that of the fluorine-18-labeled 2-deoxyglucose PET studies reported by Engel et al. (1983) (24 percent). This greater reliability may result from the superior temporal resolution of the rCBF technique.

VALIDATING THE METHOD: CASES FOR CLINICAL CORRELATION

The sensitivity of an assay must also be known to interpret results meaningfully. If we are to accept data relating to dynamic mental states as valid we must first insure that gross cerebral lesions are discernible. We have investigated a number of such cases, three of which are described below.

Case 1: Right Parietal Subdural Hematoma

A 30-year-old male subject had several years before study suffered a right parietal subdural hematoma that had been surgically evacuated. He had residual neurological deficits, including left hemiparesis and sensory loss. In analyzing structurally pathological tissue it may not be possible to clearly separate the blood flows in gray and white matter, which is assumed in using the two-compartment model. There are several blood flow measures that do not require this assumption. Figure 2 shows the results of a single study of this patient during the resting condition. Three different parameters of blood flow are depicted as percent change

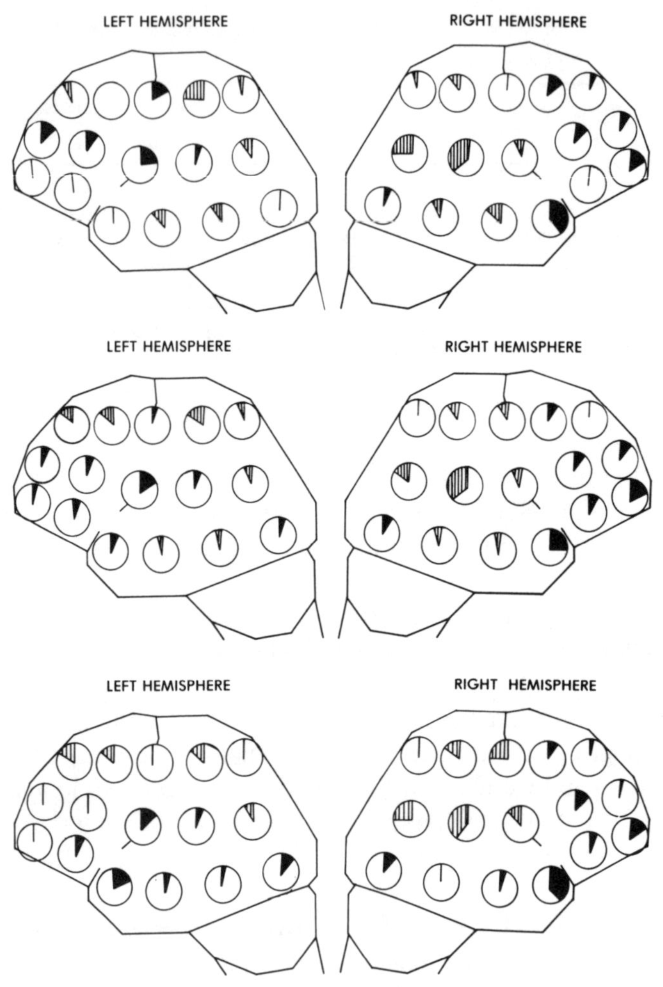

Figure 2. Resting state rCBF study of a patient status—post right parietal subdural hematoma. Values are expressed as percent change from the hemispheric mean:

$$\left(\frac{\text{Probe Value} - \text{Hemispheric Mean}}{\text{Hemispheric Mean}} \times 100 \right) \quad -15\% \quad +15\%$$

and are shown for three different blood flow parameters (see text): (top) IS, gray matter flow; (middle) ISI2, the initial slope index derived from the tangent of the clearance curve at 2.5 min; (bottom) CBF(inf), blood flow to all tissues seen by a particular probe.

from the mean: (top) IS is a noncompartmental measure derived from the initial slope (tangent) of the clearance curve at time zero and is highly correlated with the two-compartment measure of blood flow in gray matter; (middle) ISI2 is the initial slope index derived from the tangent of the clearance curve of xenon-133 at 2.5 min and correlates with both f1 and CBF(inf); (bottom) CBF(inf) represents the mean blood flow through all tissues seen by a particular probe. The figures illustrate clearly reduced flow in the right parietal area. Figure 3 depicts the same data in another fashion. Absolute values (rather than percent changes) for f1, ISI2 and CBF(inf) are indicated. The 16 probes of each hemisphere are

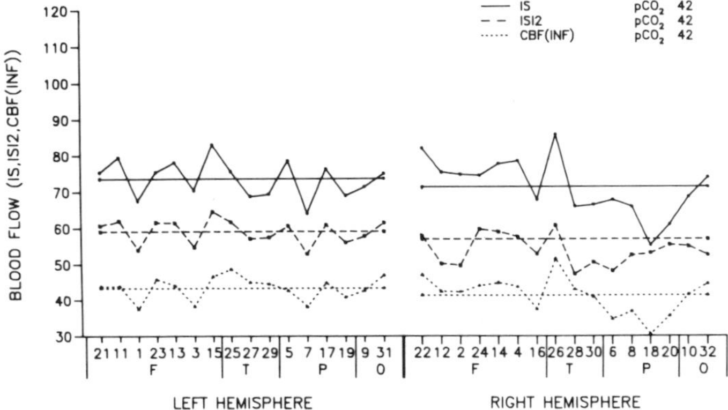

Figure 3. Resting state rCBF study of a patient status—post right parietal subdural hematoma (also see Figure 2). Absolute values are depicted with the probes of each hemisphere arranged linearly, approximately from anterior to posterior (F = frontal, T = temporal, P = parietal, O = occipital). Horizontal lines represent the hemispheric means. Three parameters are given: IS, ISI2, and CSF(inf). Note that the right parietal deficit is most apparent in the IS, gray matter flow values.

arranged roughly from anterior to posterior, and the straight lines indicate hemispheric means. Again, the deficit in right parietal activity is clear. As expected, the right parietal deficit is most apparent in the IS or flow values for gray matter.

Case 2: Fahr's Disease

A 55-year-old male subject with a 20-year history of bipolar affective disorder had been treated at various times with tricyclic antidepressants, electroconvulsant therapy, neuroleptics, and lithium. He reported increasing memory problems and decreasing productivity at work over a two-year period. Mild parkinsonian signs (bradykinesia, stooped posture, cog-wheel rigidity) appeared during the same time. An x-ray computed tomography (CT) scan revealed marked calcification of the entire basal ganglia and a portion of the frontal lobes, confirming a diagnosis of Fahr's disease (cryptogenic calcification of the basal ganglia). Figure 4 shows a rCBF study of this patient resting with eyes closed. This study is remarkable for the extent to which frontal flow is reduced in both hemispheres, consistent with the cortical calcification seen with CT.

Case 3: Moya Moya Disease

A 17-year-old boy presented in an acute catatonic state, posturing and mute, but alert. This neurological exam was unremarkable except for finding that he showed waxy flexibility and appeared to be hallucinating. He responded over a three-week course of in-patient care. One month after admission a CT scan requested by his mother revealed large bilateral frontal lobe infarction. An arteriogram confirmed a diagnosis of Moya Moya

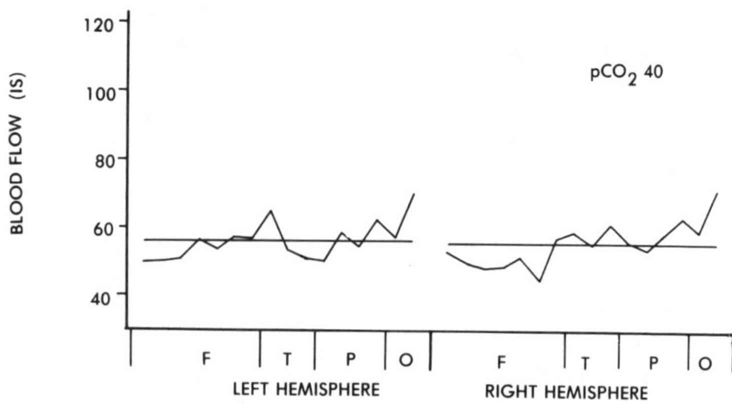

Figure 4. Resting state rCBF study of a patient with Fahr's disease (calcification of the basal ganglia and frontal lobes). Values are for gray matter flow. Note the marked decrease in frontal rCBF.

disease, a rare disorder of cerebral vasculature. One year later the subject was greatly improved, although he showed persistent memory impairment and subtle personality changes. Figure 5 shows rCBF results for this subject at rest, indicating marked bilateral "hypofrontality." These findings are consistent with the CT findings of areas of infarction, suggesting cortical hypometabolism secondary to neuronal loss.

APPLICATIONS TO RESEARCH ON SCHIZOPHRENIA

Studying the Frontal Lobes

Many of the clinical symptoms, neurological ("soft") signs, cognitive deficits, and neurophysiological patterns that are associated with schizophrenia suggest frontal lobe dysfunction. Animal and human studies indicate that the frontal lobes have a highly complex role in information processing, sequential planning, and inhibition of drive. (For a review, see Fuster 1980.) Patients with frontal lobe disease display poor judgment, inappropriate or blunted affect, bizarre and non-goal-directed behavior, and attentional deficits. Such clinical phenomena are common in schizo-

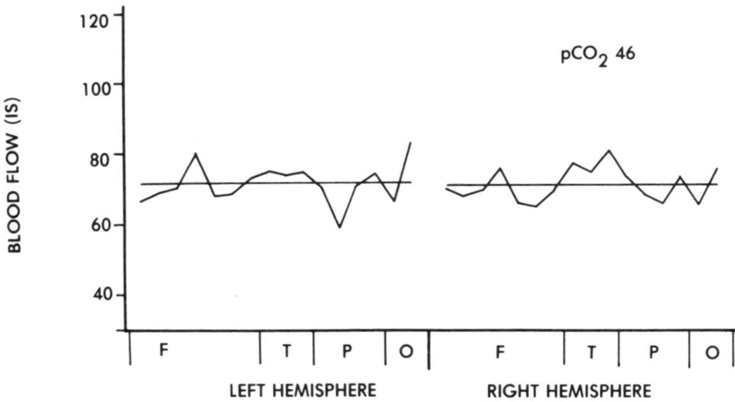

Figure 5. Gray matter flow values for a resting state rCBF study of a patient with Moya Moya disease and frontal lobe infarctions. Note the marked decrease in frontal flow.

phrenic patients, and some studies with functional brain-imaging techniques have suggested reduced frontal cortical metabolism in schizophrenic patients. These studies have been difficult to interpret however, because patients have been evaluated either at rest or while medicated.

The Wisconsin Card Sort Paradigm

Our approach has been to study unmedicated patients performing different tasks in series. One cognitive task we have employed is the Wisconsin Card Sort Test (WCS). It was selected because it has been shown to be a sensitive indicator of the integrity of the dorsolateral frontal cortex in humans (Milner 1964). Since the test is known to reveal frontal lobe damage, it seemed a good candidate for use with rCBF to detect the frontal lobe dysfunction suspected in chronic schizophrenic patients. Normal subjects might show frontal activation when performing this task, for example, while schizophrenic patients might show attenuated frontal activation or other anomalous responses.

To test this hypothesis we had subjects undergo three consecutive rCBF procedures: first, while at rest, then, in counterbalanced

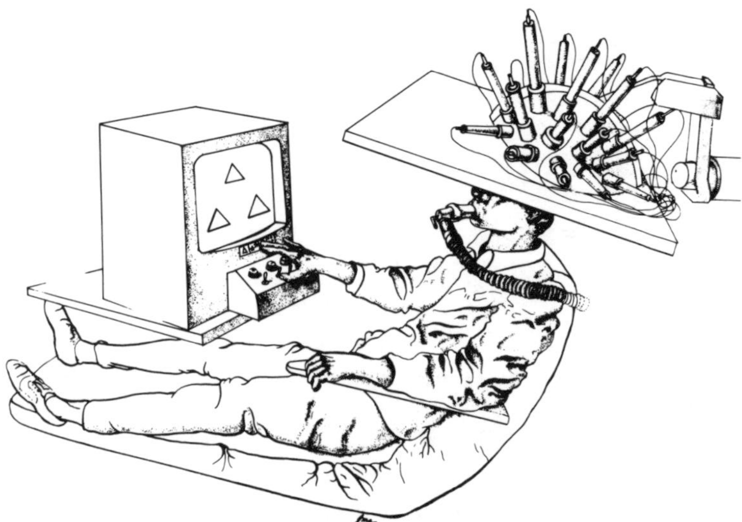

Figure 6. Procedure for performing cognitive tasks during rCBF studies.

sequence, while performing a simple numbers matching task (NM) and while taking an automated version of the WCS. The first test is always of the resting condition, primarily to acclimate the subject, but also to compare the data with that from previous studies. (Most have studied only the resting state.) In our automated WCS, subjects are shown stimulus slides of designs that differ in color, shape, and number of elements (Figure 6). They are asked to match each stimulus to one of four switches labeled with representative stimuli and must determine whether they should match by color, shape, or form solely on the basis of feedback (a green or red light) about whether each choice is correct or incorrect. Once the subject discovers the correct rule for the match and has made a series of correct responses, the rule is changed without warning, and the subject must again determine the correct solution. Responses are made with a minimum of finger movement by pressing the appropriate switch. For the NM control task subjects are shown slides of the numbers one through four which they are asked simply to match with one of four similarly labeled switches. Stimulus presentation and indication of response are carried out as in the WCS, and the subject, again, receives feedback (a red or green light) about the correctness of the response. Thus, use of the NM controls for the minimal finger movement necessary to make a response, for visual stimulation and eye scanning, and for the experience of performing a task. Differences in rCBF between NM and WCS, then, might be assumed to result largely because of the abstract reasoning necessary to perform the WCS.

This study is in the preliminary stages, but its early results are interesting. Blood flow studies of a chronic schizophrenic patient for resting, WCS, and NM paradigms are shown in Figure 7. Those of a normal volunteer appear in Figure 8. Both sets of studies are typical of their respective subject groups. The study of the chronic schizophrenic patient at rest shows a normal pattern of the frontal-to-occipital hyperfrontal gradient. During the activation procedure, however, differences arise. Our results to date, while incomplete, suggest the following: no significant difference is apparent in the ratio of frontal rCBF to parietal and occipital

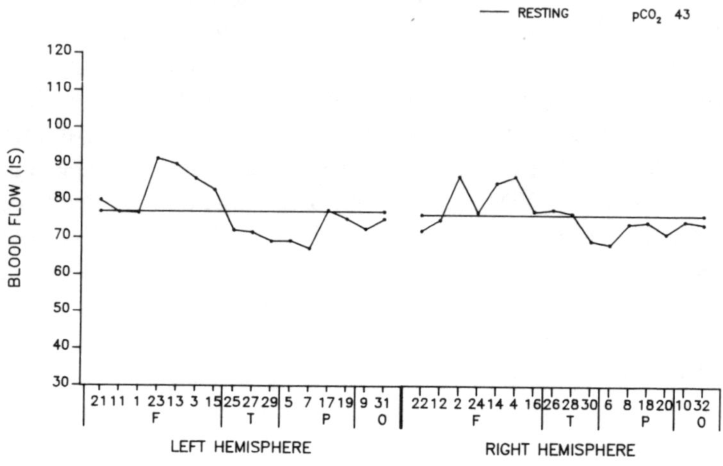

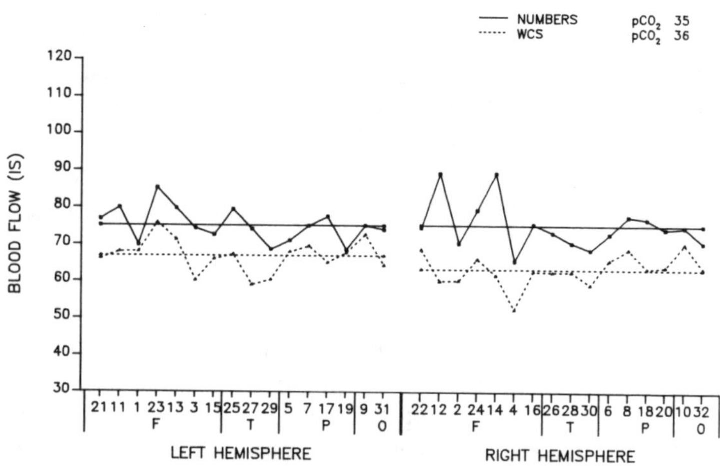

Figure 7. Results of rCBF studies of a typical chronic schizophrenic patient (gray matter flow). Note the normal "hyperfrontal" pattern at rest (top) but the reduction in CBF during the Wisconsin Card Sort paradigm (bottom).

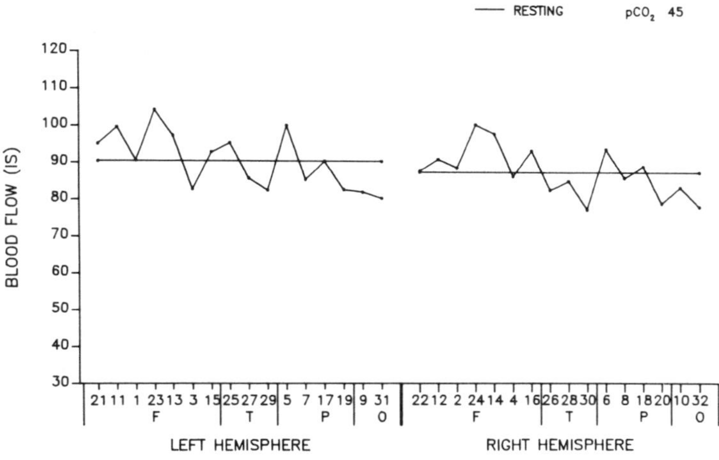

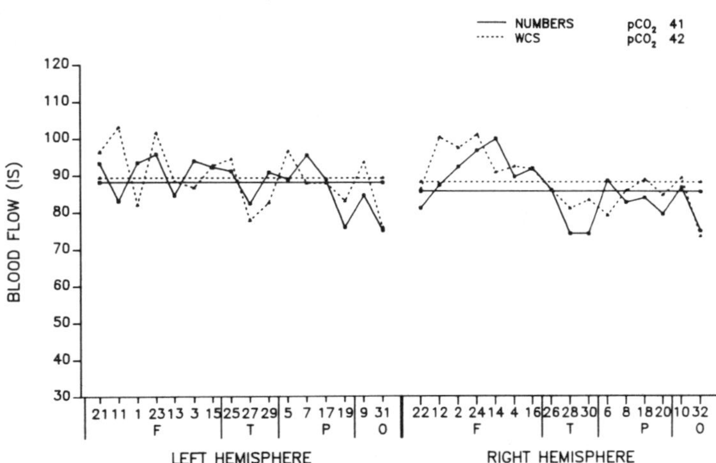

Figure 8. Results of rCBF studies of a normal volunteer (gray matter flow). Note the relative increase in frontal rCBF in both (top) resting state, and (bottom) numbers matching control task and Wisconsin Card Sort paradigm.

blood flow between the schizophrenic and control groups at rest, but during the WCS 40 to 50 percent of the chronic schizophrenics show hypofrontal function while none of the control group do. It is worth noting that the schizophrenic group makes errors on the WCS that are characteristic of frontal lobe patients, including perseverative errors and failure to maintain set.

We are pursuing our findings by studying cerebral metabolic response to this abstract reasoning task in a larger population of chronic schizophrenic patients and in a spectrum of patients with known frontal lobe abnormalities, like those mentioned in the previous section. We are also studying rCBF with subjects performing a vigilance and attention test, the continuous performance task, to evaluate how specifically the findings are related to frontal cognitive demand.

CONCLUSIONS

The promise of functional brain-imaging techniques like rCBF is that brain-behavior relations can be studied while the subject is alert and actively engaged in different sorts of psychological "activation" (for example, in different cognitive and mood states). Biological concomitants of higher cognitive functions both in normal and pathological conditions may thus be investigated.

rCBF measurement by inhalation of xenon-133 is in many ways particularly well-suited to this formidable task, but it should not be considered or applied without a full understanding of its limits and strengths. More important, the use of rCBF is not an end in itself. It is a promising tool, but still an imperfect one, for attempting to localize and characterize mental phenomena in the living human brain. We have described some interesting preliminary results from an ongoing study of schizophrenia. They suggest this disorder is related to a dysfunction in dorsolateral frontal cortical activation.

References

Deshmukh VD, Meyer JS: Noninvasive Measurement of Regional Cerebral Blood Flow in Man. New York, Spectrum Publications, 1978

Engel J Jr, Kuhl DE, Phelps ME, et al: Local cerebral metabolism during partial seizures. Neurology 33:400–413, 1983

Franzen G, Ingvar DH: Abnormal distribution of cerebral activity in chronic schizophrenia. J Psychiatr Res 12:199–214, 1975

Fuster J: The Prefrontal Cortex. New York, Raven Press, 1980

Ingvar DH: Functional landscapes of the dominant hemisphere. Brain Res 107:181–197, 1976

Ingvar DH, Franzen G: Abnormalities of cerebral blood distribution in patients with chronic schizophrenia. Acta Psychiatr Scand 50:425–462, 1974

Ingvar DH, Conqvist R, Ekberg K, et al: Normal values of regional cerebral blood flow in man including flow and weight estimates of gray and white matter. Acta Neurol Scand [Supp] 14:72–78, 1965

Kety SS, Schmidt CF: The determination of cerebral blood flow in man by use of nitrous oxide in low concentrations. Am J Physiol 143:53–66, 1945

Kety SS, Woodford RB, Harvard MH, et al: Cerebral blood flow and metabolism in schizophrenia: effects of barbiturate seminarcosis, insulin coma and electroshock. Am J Psychiatry 104:765–770, 1948

Mallet BL, Veall N: Measurement of regional cerebral clearance rates in man using ^{133}xenon inhalation and extracranial recording. Clin Sci 29:124–135, 1965

Matthew RJ, Duncan GC, Weiman ML, et al: Regional cerebral blood flow in schizophrenia. Arch Gen Psychiatry 39:1121–1124, 1982

Mazziotta JC, Phelps ME, Carson RE, et al: Tomographic mapping of human cerebral metabolism: sensory deprivation. Ann Neurol 12:435–444, 1982

Milner B: Some effects of frontal lobectomy in man, in The Frontal Granular Cortex and Behavior. Edited by Warren JM, Akert K. New York, McGraw-Hill, 1964

Obrist WD, Wilkinson WE: The non-invasive Xe^{133} method: evaluation of CBF indices, in Cerebral Circulation. Edited by Bes A, Geraud G. Amsterdam, Elsevier North-Holland, 1980

Obrist WD, Thompson HK, Wang HS, et al: A simplified procedure for determining fast compartment rCBF by ^{133}xenon inhalation, in Brain and Blood Flow. Edited by Russell RWR. London, Pitman Publishing Company, 1971

Obrist WD, Thompson HK, Wang HS, et al: Regional cerebral blood flow estimated by $xenon^{133}$ inhalation. Stroke 6:245–256, 1975

Risberg J, Ali Z, Wilson EM, et al: Regional cerebral blood flow by ^{133}xenon inhalation. Stroke 6:142–148, 1975

US Nuclear Regulatory Commission, Title 10, Chapter 1, CFR Part 19, Notices, Instructions and Reports to Workers, Inspections; Part 20, Standards for Protection Against Radiation; Part 30, Rules of General Applicability to Licensing of Byproduct Material

US Nuclear Regulatory Commission, Title 10, Chapter 1, CFR, Part 35, Human Uses of Byproduct Material

Veall N, Mallett BL: Regional cerebral blood flow determination by ^{133}xenon inhalation and external recording: the effect of arterial recirculation. Clin Sci 30:353–369, 1966

4

Regional Cerebral Blood Flow in Psychiatry: The Resting and Activated Brains of Schizophrenic Patients

Raquel E. Gur, M.D., Ph.D.

4

Regional Cerebral Blood Flow in Psychiatry: The Resting and Activated Brains of Schizophrenic Patients

The investigation of regional brain functioning in schizophrenia has been based on behavioral techniques. Although results are sometimes inconsistent, the behavioral observations suggest left hemispheric dysfunction (Flor-Henry 1976; Gur 1977, 1978; Wexler 1980) and left hemispheric overactivation (Gur 1978; Schweitzer et al. 1978). Recent developments in neuroimaging technology make possible major refinements in assessing regional brain function. Both anatomical and physiological information can now be used to study regional brain involvement in psychiatric disorders. This chapter describes the application of one method—the xenon-133 technique for measuring regional cerebral blood flow (rCBF)—in studying the resting and activated brains of schizophrenic patients.

REGIONAL CEREBRAL BLOOD FLOW IN SCHIZOPHRENIA

The xenon-133 techniques stem from Kety and Schmidt's nitrous oxide method for determining whole brain cerebral blood flow (CBF) (Kety and Schmidt 1945, 1948). Schizophrenics and normals show no consistent differences in whole brain CBF (Kety et al. 1948; Wilson et al. 1952; Gordan et al. 1955; Della Porta et al. 1964;

Hoyer and Oesterreich 1975). Initial studies of rCBF used intracarotid injection, which can assess only one hemisphere at a time. Ingvar and Franzen (1974a, 1974b) reported lower frontal flows in elderly chronic schizophrenics.

Bilateral rCBF measurements were enabled by the development of the xenon-133 inhalation technique (Obrist et al. 1975; Risberg et al. 1975a). A trace amount of the gas is inhaled and its clearance from the brain is measured by extracranial scintillation detectors. Clearance is a function of blood flow in two main compartments: well-perfused, fast-clearing tissue, primarily gray matter; and less perfused, slow-clearing tissue, primarily white matter. The rCBF indices are calculated from these clearance rates (Obrist and Wilkinson 1979).

Three studies have been published on bilateral resting rCBF in schizophrenics. Mathew et al (1981), using a "modified" Initial Slope Index (ISI) of blood flow (Risberg et al. 1975a), reported lower right hemispheric flows in a sample of 6 chronic schizophrenics compared to 6 normals. In a second study (Mathew et al. 1982), also using the ISI, decreased flows were reported globally in a sample of 23 schizophrenics (mean ISI = 53.4) compared to 18 controls (mean ISI = 58.6). In this study, however, schizophrenics had significantly lower PCO_2 levels. When the standard correction of rCBF for PCO_2 is applied (3 percent per 1 mm Hg of change in PCO_2), the corrected values of rCBF for schizophrenics (mean ISI = 57.9) do not differ from those for controls.

Ariel et al. (1983) reported decreased resting rCBF in all brain regions in a sample of 29 schizophrenics compared to 22 controls. It is noteworthy that 11 patients had a history of alcohol abuse and 12 reported street drug use, although none qualified for a DSM-III diagnosis of abuse. In addition, the educational level of schizophrenics was lower (mean 11 years, range 3 to 16 years) than that of controls (mean 16.6 years, range 12 to 20 years). Although there is no direct evidence that rCBF values and educational level correlate, a number of factors associated with educational level may correlate with rCBF. Ariel et al. (1983) found no significant correlations between educational level and rCBF values for each group. Nevertheless, the range of education represented is rather narrow within groups and the possibility of an overall correlation between education and rCBF was not examined.

In all studies reporting reduced rCBF values in schizophrenics there was a higher proportion of men in the patient groups, and sex differences were not examined. In view of the documented sex differences in rCBF values, with women having higher flows (Gur et al. 1982), the effects of diagnosis may be confounded with sex in such studies.

Gur and colleagues (1983) found no difference in resting rCBF between medicated schizophrenics and controls matched for age, sex, and education. Significant differences between patients and controls were noted in regional blood flow changes during cognitive tasks.

ACTIVATED rCBF

Gur et al. (1983) studied a sample of 15 medicated schizophrenics, 7 men and 8 women. Patients were diagnosed by DSM-III criteria and satisfied the Research Diagnostic Criteria (RDC) for the diagnosis. All patients were right-handed. rCBF was measured using Obrist's xenon-133 inhalation technique. The clearance rates were measured with 16 NaI scintillation detectors, placed over 8 homotopic regions in the left and right hemispheres. The detector arrangement is shown in Figure 1.

The rCBF measurements were performed under three standardized conditions, in random, counterbalanced order: while the subject rested, with eyes open, with ambient noise kept to a minimum, and with the subject instructed to relax, stay quiet, and not fall asleep; while the subject performed a verbal task, solving verbal analogies such as those used in the Scholastic Aptitude Test; and while the subject performed a spatial task, an adaptation of Benton and colleagues' (1975) Line Orientation Test. Motor response was equal for both tasks: pointing a light beam with both hands to the correct answer. These task conditions had produced reliable increases in rCBF values in a sample of 62 undergraduate volunteers. The laterality of change was affected by the task, with greater left hemispheric increase for the verbal task and greater right hemispheric increase for the spatial task (Gur et al. 1982). The medicated schizophrenics were compared to a new sample of 25 normal volunteers who were matched for sex, age, and education. As indicated above, no resting rCBF differences were obtained between patients and controls. Furthermore, both groups showed comparable rCBF increases during the cognitive tasks. Unlike controls, however, patients showed no lateralized effects in completing verbal analogies and greater left hemispheric increase for the spatial task. This pattern is distinctly different from the normal rCBF response to cognitive activation tasks. The significant Diagnosis $\times$ Sex $\times$ Task $\times$ Hemisphere interaction is illustrated in Figure 2.

The finding was interpreted as consistent with the hypothesized left hemispheric relative overactivation in schizophrenia. The study does not strongly support the hypothesis, however,

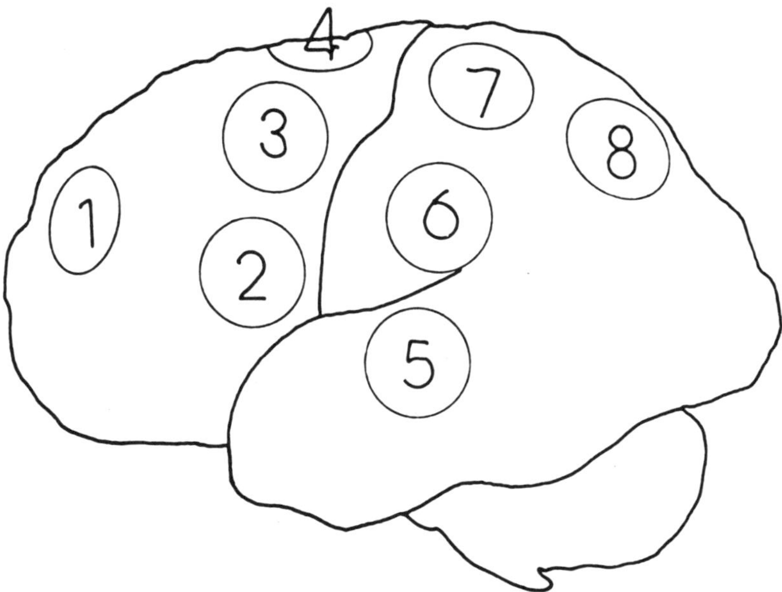

Figure 1. Detector placement. Curvature of circles reflects detector orientation (from Gur et al. 1983).

since lateralized abnormalities in schizophrenics were pronounced only during the spatial task. There is some evidence that neuroleptics attenuate behavioral indicators of lateralized abnormalities in schizophrenia (Myslobodsky and Weiner 1976; Mintz et al. 1982). It can therefore be expected that lateralized abnormalities may be more pronounced in unmedicated schizophrenics.

A sample of 19 unmedicated schizophrenics (11 men, 8 women) was compared to 19 matched controls (Gur et al., manuscript submitted for publication). The tasks and conditions were identical to the previous study. As expected, laterality effects were enhanced in unmedicated patients. In contrast to medicated schizophrenics, who showed no abnormalities in resting rCBF, unmedicated schizophrenics showed significant lateralized ab-

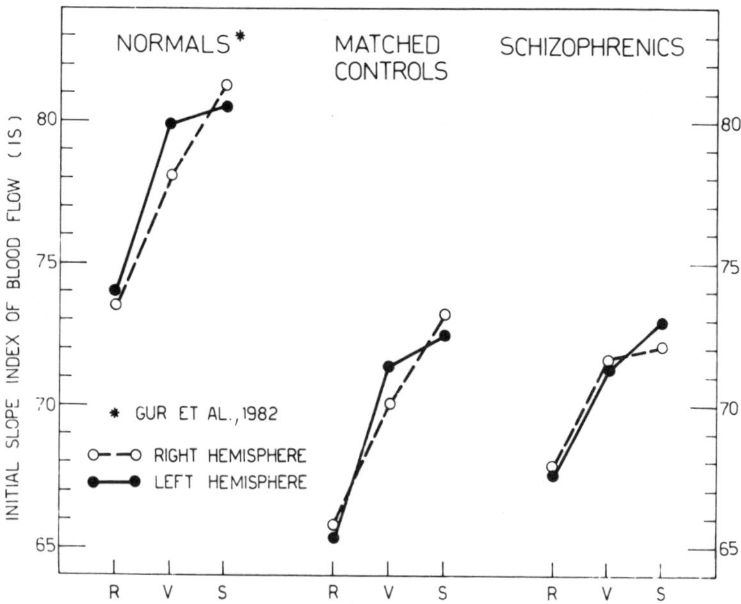

Figure 2.   Regional cerebral blood flow in each hemisphere of schizophrenic subjects and matched controls when resting (R), solving verbal analogies (V), and performing a spatial task (S). Values for controls on the far left are from Gur et al. (1982), a study of young college undergraduates. These data are presented for comparison with those on generally older and less educated controls matched for the schizophrenic subjects (from Gur et al. 1983).

normalities in this condition. The patients did not differ from controls in overall resting flows, but there was a Diagnosis $\times$ Hemisphere interaction. Resting flows were equal in the two hemispheres for controls, as in other studies (Risberg et al. 1975a; Prohovnik et al. 1980; Gur and Reivich 1980; Gur et al. 1982). They were higher in the left hemisphere for schizophrenics. Thus, the hypothesized left hemispheric overactivation in schizophrenia was observed in the resting condition. Analysis of flows during activation conditions indicated lateralized abnormalities as well, further supporting the hypothesis of increased left hemispheric activity. Every deviation of hemispheric flows in unmedicated schizophrenics compared to controls was toward higher rCBF in the left hemisphere of schizophrenics.

The rCBF also allowed study of anterior-posterior regional brain abnormalities in schizophrenics. Hypofrontal resting flows were reported in schizophrenics (Ingvar and Franzen 1974b). The analysis of variance in the Gur et al. study of unmedicated schizophrenics (manuscript submitted for publication) did not show a significant Diagnosis $\times$ Anterior-Posterior interaction for the resting rCBF. There was only a marginally significant interaction of Diagnosis $\times$ Anterior-Posterior $\times$ Probe location, and this indicated higher than normal flows in schizophrenics in the most anterior and the most posterior detector locations.

A significant Task $\times$ Diagnosis $\times$ Sex $\times$ Hemisphere $\times$ Anterior-Posterior indicated that all factors examined in the study contributed to rCBF abnormalities in schizophrenia. The analysis revealed that a number of features distinguished schizophrenics from controls, against a background of common features. Common features were higher flows in anterior regions, higher flows in females, and higher flows during cognitive activity. Schizophrenic males were distinguished by unusual activity in the precentral region. They showed higher flows in the left compared to the right hemisphere during both rest and the verbal task. Furthermore, unlike controls, who had the highest overall flows during the spatial task, and higher in the right than the left hemisphere for that task, schizophrenics had lower flows during the spatial than during the verbal task, and their flows were equal for the two hemispheres. Female schizophrenics differed from female controls in both anterior and posterior regions. In anterior regions, they differed by showing less increase during the spatial task. In the posterior regions, normals had the same flows for resting, higher flows in the left hemisphere for the verbal task, and higher flows in the right hemisphere for the spatial task. Schizophrenics had higher left hemisphere flows for all three conditions. Thus, all differences were toward higher left hemisphere flows in schizophrenics compared to controls, and the effects were more marked for anterior regions in males and for posterior regions in females.

THE EFFECTS OF NEUROLEPTICS

The effects of antipsychotic medication have not been examined systematically with rCBF. Mathew et al. (1982) reported no differences in resting rCBF between medicated schizophrenics ($N = 13$) and patients who had undergone a one-week period without drugs ($N = 9$). Likewise, Ariel et al. (1983) found no correlations between medication levels and rCBF. However, of the few studies that have tested the effects of neuroleptic medication on lateralized brain function, Mintz et al. (1982) found lateralized effects on visual evoked potentials. This suggests that neuroleptic medication improves regional brain functioning in schizophrenics.

In comparing the medicated and unmedicated schizophrenics studied by Gur et al. (manuscript submitted for publication), a significant effect of medication was found in resting rCBF. The effect was different in men and in women. Medicated males in anterior regions showed increased right hemispheric resting flows and decreased left hemispheric flows compared to unmedicated schizophrenic males. In posterior regions, a bilateral increase in rCBF was associated with medication, and the increase was greater in the right hemisphere. In females, the effect of medication was a bilateral increase in flows, both anterior and posterior, and the flows in medicated patients became more symmetric. No additional effects of medication were found when activated flows were considered in the analysis.

It is noteworthy that these between-group comparisons may mask more subtle effects of medication that may be detected when the same patients are studied before and after medication. Furthermore, both groups of patients were studied in the acute phase, and the effects of medication on symptomatology had not been stabilized at the time of study for the medicated patients. This may have led to underestimating the effects of medication. On the other hand, the effects that have been obtained may not be confounded by behavioral changes, and they can be taken as a conservative estimate of the pure effects of medication. The results suggest the following conclusions: Neuroleptic medication produces lateralized rCBF changes. The effects in males are toward relatively increased right hemispheric flows. In females, neuroleptic medication produces an overall increase in flow and greater symmetry in flow. Medication affects resting flows, and no effects were observed on rCBF reactivity to stimulation with cognitive tasks.

SUMMARY

The use of isotopic techniques to study regional brain activity in psychiatric disorders is just now beginning. This chapter described the use of the xenon-133 technique for measuring regional cerebral blood flow in schizophrenic patients. Initial studies have reported inconsistent data, but they did not control for sex and effects of medication. Furthermore, they examined only resting flows. In a study comparing medicated schizophrenics to matched controls, no differences between patients and controls were found in resting rCBF. Flows measured during "activation" with cognitive tasks revealed abnormalities in hemispheric changes during task performance. Specifically, schizophrenics showed overactivation of the left hemisphere compared to controls for the spatial task. In a subsequent study of unmedicated schizophrenics, once again, no overall differences in resting rCBF were found in comparison to matched controls. There were hemispheric differences in resting rCBF, however, with controls showing symmetric flows while schizophrenics had higher left hemispheric flows. Activated flows likewise showed left hemispheric overactivation in schizophrenic subjects, and the effects were more pronounced in the unmedicated group. Direct comparisons of medicated and unmedicated patients suggested that the effects of medication are different for males and females in the anterior and posterior regions. In general, medication increased right hemispheric flows. The results support the hypothesis of left hemispheric overactivation in schizophrenia. They also suggest the utility of further systematic examination of the effects of activation, medication, sex, and the anterior-posterior dimension as experimental factors. Such investigations are possible with isotopic methods for measuring regional brain activity.

References

Ariel RN, Golden CJ, Berg RA, et al: Regional cerebral blood flow in schizophrenics. Arch Gen Psychiatry 40:258–263, 1983

Benton AL, Varney NR, des Hamsher K: Judgment of Line Orientation. Iowa City, University of Iowa Hospitals, 1975

Della Porta P, Maiolo AT, Negri VU, et al: Cerebral blood flow and metabolism in therapeutic insulin coma. Metabolism 13:131–140, 1964

Flor-Henry P: Lateralized temporal-limbic dysfunction and psychopathology. Ann NY Acad Sci 280:777–795, 1976

Gordan GS, Esters FM, Adams JE, et al: Cerebral oxygen uptake in chronic schizophrenic reaction. Archives of Neurology and Psychiatry 73:544–545, 1955

Gur RC, Reivich M: Cognitive task effects on hemispheric blood flow in humans. Brain Lang 9:78–93, 1980

Gur RC, Gur RE, Obrist WD, et al: Sex and handedness differences in cerebral blood flow during rest and cognitive activity. Science 217:659–661, 1982

Gur RE: Motoric laterality imbalance in schizophrenia: a possible concomitant of left hemisphere dysfunction. Arch Gen Psychiatry 34:33–37, 1977

Gur RE: Left hemisphere dysfunction and left hemisphere overactivation in schizophrenia. J Abnorm Psychol 87:225–238, 1978

Gur RE, Skolnick BE, Gur RC, et al: Brain function in psychiatric disorders, I: Regional cerebral blood flow in medicated schizophrenics. Arch Gen Psychiatry 40:1250–1254, 1983

Gur RE, Gur RC, Skolnick BE, et al: Brain function in psychiatric disorders, III: regional cerebral blood flow in unmedicated schizophrenics. Manuscript submitted for publication

Hoyer S, Oesterreich K: Blood flow and oxidative metabolism of the brain in patients with schizophrenia. Psychiatr Clin 8:304–313, 1975

Ingvar DH, Franzen G: Distribution of cerebral activity in chronic schizophrenia. Lancet 2:1484–1486, 1974a

Ingvar DH, Franzen G: Abnormalities of cerebral blood flow distribution in patients with chronic schizophrenia. Acta Psychiatr Scand 50:425–462, 1974b

Kety SS, Schmidt CF: The determination of cerebral blood flow in man by the use of nitrous oxide in low concentrations. Am J Physiol 143:53–66, 1945

Kety SS, Schmidt CF: The nitrous oxide method for the quantitative determination of cerebral blood flow in man: theory, procedure and normal values. J Clin Invest 27:476–483, 1948

Kety SS, Woodford RB, Harmel MH, et al: Cerebral blood flow and metabolism in schizophrenia. The effects of barbiturate, semi-narcosis, insulin coma and electroshock. Am J Psychiatry 104:765–770, 1948

Mathew RJ, Meyer JS, Francis DJ, et al: Regional cerebral blood flow in schizophrenia: a preliminary report. Am J Psychiatry 138:112–113, 1981

Mathew RJ, Duncan GC, Weinman ML, et al: Regional cerebral blood flow in schizophrenia. Arch Gen Psychiatry 39:1121–1124, 1982

Mintz M, Tomer R, Myslobodsky MS: Neuroleptic-induced lateral asymmetry of visual evoked potentials in schizophrenia. Biol Psychiatry 17:815–828, 1982

Myslobodsky MS, Weiner M: Pharmacologic implications of hemispheric asymmetry. Life Sci 19:1467–1478, 1976

Obrist WD, Wilkinson WE: The non-invasive Xe-133 method: evaluation of CBF indices, in Cerebral Circulation. Edited by Bes A, Geraud G. Elsevier, North Holland, 1979

Obrist WD, Thompson HK, Wang HS, et al: Regional cerebral blood flow estimated by 133-Xe inhalation. Stroke 6:245–256, 1975

Prohovnik I, Hakansson K, Risberg J: Observations on the functional significance of regional cerebral blood flow in "resting" normal subjects. Neuropsychologia 18:203–217, 1980

Risberg J, Halsey JH, Wills EL, et al: Hemispheric specialization in normal man studied by bilateral measurement of the regional cerebral blood flow—a study with the 133-Xe inhalation technique. Brain 98:511–524, 1975a

Risberg J, Ali Z, Wilson EM, et al: Regional cerebral blood flow by 133 xenon inhalation. Stroke 6:142–148, 1975b

Schweitzer L, Becker E, Welsh H: Abnormalities of cerebral lateralization in schizophrenic patients. Arch Gen Psychiatry 35:982–985, 1978

Wexler BE: Cerebral laterality and psychiatry: a review of the literature. Am J Psychiatry 137:279–291, 1980

Wilson WP, Schieve JF, Scheinberg P: Effect of series of electric shock treatments on cerebral blood flow and metabolism. Archives of Neurology and Psychiatry 68:651–654, 1952

5

Brain Electrical Activity Mapping (BEAM) in Psychiatry

John M. Morihisa, M.D.
Frank H. Duffy, M.D.
Richard Jed Wyatt, M.D.

5

Brain Electrical Activity Mapping (BEAM) in Psychiatry

The history of computerized electroencephalographic (EEG) and evoked potential studies in psychiatry is unique compared to that of the other brain-imaging techniques described in this book. The first EEG in man was recorded in 1929 by a psychiatrist, Hans Berger, who hoped that EEG studies would elucidate the underlying cause of mental disease. From the very beginning electrophysiological studies of the brain were integrally bound up with the technology of the times. As new scientific and engineering achievements became available, they were applied to the various perplexing problems of psychophysiological research. With new technical advances, what began as novel research became routine clinical practice in many applications from investigating and classifying the epilepsies to evaluating brain death. These developments raised the expectation that such techniques might unlock the secrets of the pathophysiology of major psychotic disorders. Results have fallen considerably short of the expectation. Yet with each advance in technology and theory another veil is lifted from the mysteries of the electrical activity of the brain. Although results have fallen short of Berger's early hopes, EEG studies in psychiatry continue to grow from the single-lead scalp recordings of Berger's time to 20- and 32-channel recordings of the 1980s, to sleep studies (Dement and Fisher 1963; Rechtschaffen et al. 1964; Gillin et al. 1972; Kupfer et al. 1973) telemetry (Stevens and Livermore 1982), evoked potential studies (Gershon and Buchsbaum 1977; Shagass et al. 1979, 1980), and spectral analysis (Itil et al. 1972). Most recently, attempts have been made to use computers and new advances in solid state electronics to manage the great quantities of data produced by multiple-lead EEG and evoked potential recordings. As we enter this new phase of electrophysiological research we must be careful to use these highly sophisticated techniques as tools and not be smothered in the profusion of information that they generate. This will be an issue for all the brain-imaging approaches now being introduced to medicine. One aim of this book has been to familiarize the clinician with several different brain-imaging approaches now being applied in psychiatry, both to present the newest findings and to provide a critical framework for evaluating these findings and techniques before they are assimilated for clinical use. In our final case example we examine the technique of brain electrical activity mapping (BEAM) as it is used to generate color maps of electrical activity in schizophrenic patients and normal controls. We focus here on BEAM data that are pertinent to the findings of other brain-imaging techniques. A more extensive examination of BEAM data on schizophrenic patients is presented elsewhere (Morihisa et al. 1983a).

METHODOLOGY

Subjects

The subjects were chronic schizophrenic inpatients who fulfilled DSM III (American Psychiatric Association 1980) criteria and Research Diagnostic Criteria (Spitzer et al. 1977). Eleven patients had been drug-free for at least four weeks and 14 patients had been medicated for at least four weeks on a standard dose of haloperidol (0.4 mg/kg). The control group consisted of 11 normal subjects with no history of psychiatric or neurological abnormality. Patients were not significantly different from controls in age, gender, or handedness.

Data Recording

In 1979 Duffy and colleagues extended the pioneering work of others by developing a computerized technique to condense and summarize EEG and evoked potential data in the form of color maps. In this technique, 25 gold cup electrodes (20 data electrodes, 2 eye electrodes, 1 ground electrode, and 2 ear reference electrodes) are applied to the scalp with collodion according to the standard international 10–20 system of placement (Figure 1). The electrical activity of the brain from each of the 20 data electrodes is then amplified through a 20-channel polygraph (Grass 78) and then recorded on a 28-channel FM analog tape recorder (Honeywell 5600 E). The data are then analyzed by a computer (DEC PDP 11-60). EEG segments containing artifacts are eliminated prior to spectral analysis by visual inspection of each segment. This process is facilitated by using data from electrodes placed to monitor eye movement.

Spectral Analysis

The signals are tightly filtered at 24 dB per octave using active

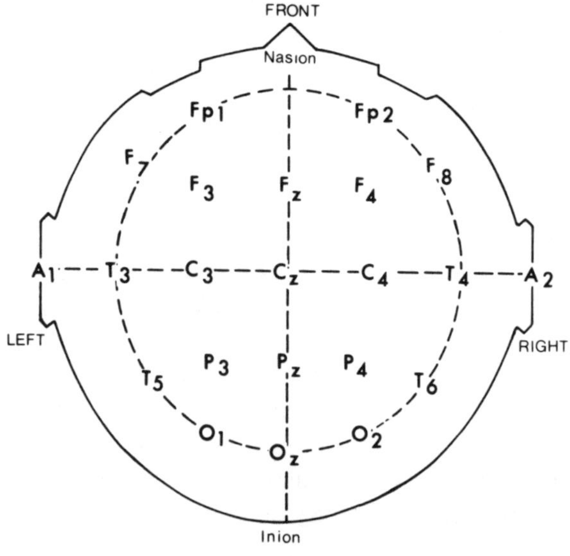

Figure 1. The electrode placements used in brain electrical activity mapping are depicted on an outline of the head as if looking down at the top of the head with nose at top and ears to left and right.

Butterworth filters in order to avoid 60-Hz noise (from other electrical devices) and artifacts of muscle activity. Prior to computer analysis all raw EEG data, including those from eye channels, were visually inspected. All EEG data reflecting eye blinks, eye movements, muscle potentials, artifacts of movement, or 60-Hz interference are then eliminated. The process of eliminating contaminated data is done blind to diagnosis. A spectral analysis from 0 to 32 Hz is then performed on the data using the Fast Fourier Transform technique, which provides a breakdown of the relative distribution of high and low frequencies in brain electrical activity. Then the amount of energy at each electrode is determined for the EEG bands of delta, theta, alpha, and beta. These data may then be used to create maps of brain electrical activity. For each of these frequency ranges, 20 values (one for each electrode) are obtained.

Evoked Potentials

In order to generate simple visual evoked potentials each subject is presented flashes of light from a photic stimulator (Grass PS-2) that is placed 16 cm in front of the subject. These light flashes are presented in a random manner. A total of 525 stimuli are presented. After each stimulus, evoked potentials of 512 msec are recorded for analysis. The program that averages the evoked potentials rejects segments of high voltage movement artifact. For this process the background polygraphic record obtained during stimulation is inspected and the rejection level is individually optimized for each subject. Then a determination is made for each electrode site of the average evoked potential voltage over the 512 msec. These 20 evoked potentials may be used for topographic mapping.

Formation of Color Maps

Topographic color maps may now be created from the 20 spectra (energy in an EEG band) or 20 evoked potentials (energy at any 4-msec period after the stimulus). The 20 values are distributed over a graphic outline of the head in the relative positions assigned by the 10–20 system of electrode placement. A 64 × 64 matrix is then overlaid on this field of 20 values. This defines 4,096 picture elements (pixels) that comprise the brain electrical activity map. Through linear interpolation of the three nearest electrode sites, each pixel is assigned a value. This facilitates the presentation of certain aspects of the data but also introduces an averaging effect on gradients between different electrodes. One must therefore be careful to avoid interpretations that rely only on distinctions based on map boundaries between electrode points as they represent an averaged gradient. Caution should also be applied in interpreting maps generated by other two-dimensional approaches such as cerebral blood flow.

A color scale is fitted to the pixel values so that each color represents a range of voltages. It is important to note that in "fitting" a color scale to the data it is possible to highlight certain findings or obscure others. Both the investigator and the reader should be cautious in interpreting the meaning of these color maps, as in interpreting the results of all the brain-imaging techniques that employ maps to display data. To overcome some of the difficulties that are inherent in the subjective interpretation of electrical activity maps, a statistical technique, significance probability mapping, is used.

Significance Probability Mapping

The technique of significance probability mapping is used to delineate topographic regions where two clinical populations differ from one another (Duffy et al. 1981). This process uses a parametric statistical test (Student's t-test) of the difference between group means, with set significance levels, to demonstrate areas of regional difference between schizophrenic patient groups and control groups. The difference is presented in the form of a color map. Thus, regional group differences are depicted so to be easily comprehended. Significance probability mapping is a form of exploratory data analysis (Tukey 1977) and is not used to address the overall significance of group differences. This issue has been addressed elsewhere (Morihisa et al. 1983a) using multivariate discriminant analysis. In other words, the statistical technique of significance probability mapping is best used when developing

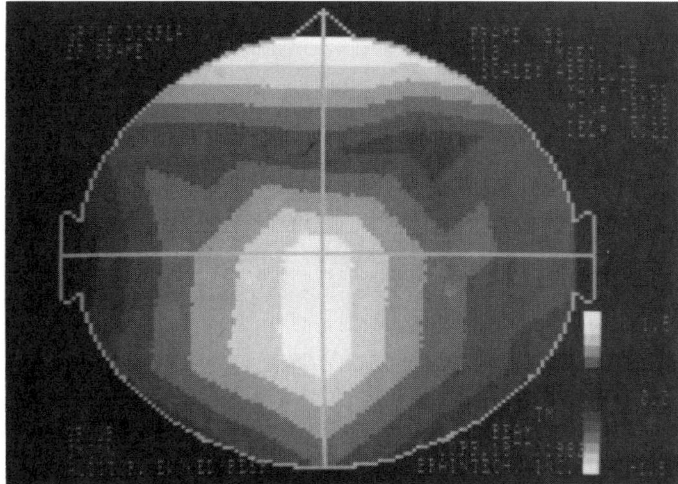

Figure 2. A brain electrical activity map of part of an evoked potential summarizing results from 11 control subjects, looking down on the head with nose at top. White shades designate highest electrical activity. Figures 2 through 4 demonstrate how a significance probability map (SPM) is created. Figures 2 through 4 use data from a separate report of a case study of schizophrenia and are reprinted from Morihisa et al. (1982).

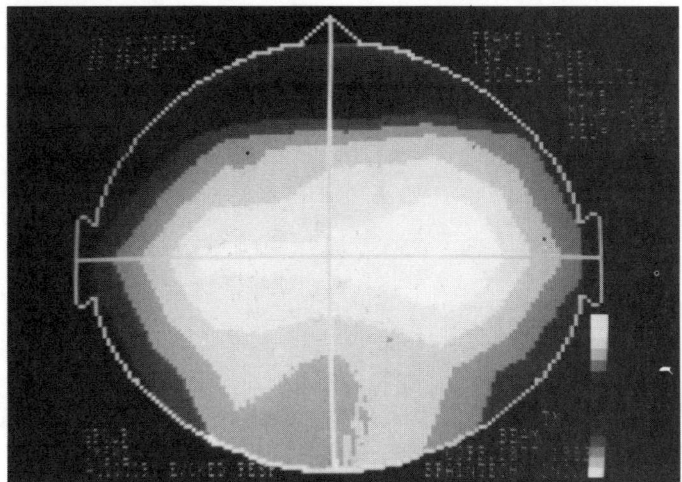

Figure 3. A brain electrical activity map of the same part of an evoked potential summarizing results from 15 schizophrenic subjects.

hypotheses rather than in testing them. The process of creating a significance probability map is demonstrated in Figures 2 through 4.

RESULTS

Spectral Analysis

Both medicated and unmedicated schizophrenic patients demonstrated increased bilateral EEG delta activity when compared to control subjects. The significance probability maps rendered visible between-group differences, which were somewhat more marked in frontal regions, that were seen over the entire cortical surface (Figure 5). Both schizophrenic groups demonstrated similar regional differences in delta activity compared to controls. Medicated schizophrenic patients showed less difference in delta activity than the unmedicated group compared to controls.

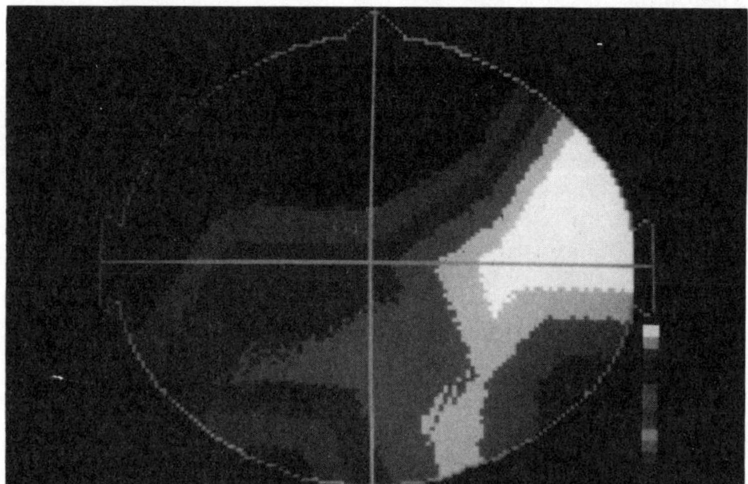

Figure 4. A significance probability map that depicts statistical relations between the two groups represented in Figures 2 and 3. White shades designate greatest regional differences between groups. Note the marked regional difference.

For fast beta activity (beta 5), posterior regions of group difference were delineated by significance probability mapping for unmedicated schizophrenic patients in the eyes open state. The greatest regional difference was noted in the left temporal-parietal area (Figure 6). Difference in beta activity in this region was associated with a relatively increased coefficient of variation, suggesting that the schizophrenic group exhibited greater beta variability.

Evoked Potentials

For the visual evoked potential, significance probability maps delineated a regional difference in the left parietal region, which occurred at 448 msec after the flash of light and persisted for over

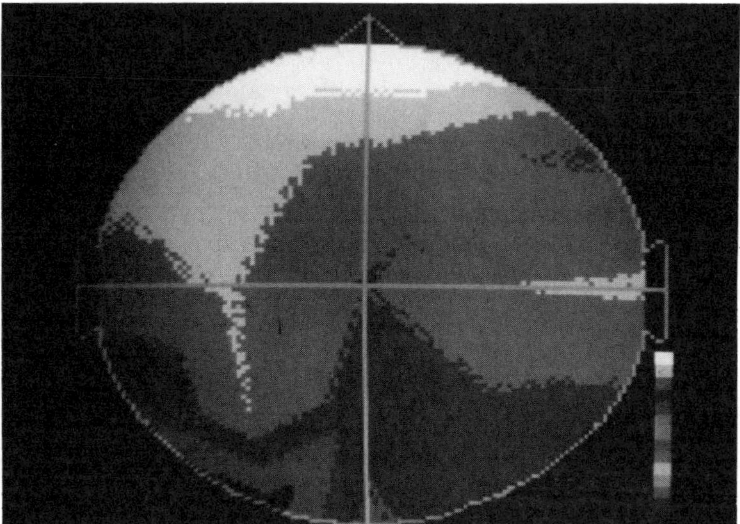

Figure 5. Significance probability map comparing delta activity of schizophrenic patients (medicated and unmedicated) with normal controls. The color scale represents increasing gradations of regional difference, white delineates areas of greatest delta difference. Schizophrenic patients demonstrated more delta activity than normals over all cortical areas. This difference was most marked in frontal regions. This figure combines the data for the medicated and unmedicated schizophrenic patients and compares it to normal controls. This map uses subject groups described in a study by Morihisa et al. (1983b).

20 msec and which represented augmented electrical activity in this region for schizophrenic patients (Figure 7).

DISCUSSION

The finding of a large bilateral increase in EEG delta activity in schizophrenic patients is consistent with one of the first applications of analog computer power spectral analysis. Itil et al. (1972) reported that schizophrenic patients as a group demonstrated a greater amount of slow (delta) activity. Using EEG telemetry, Stevens (1982) also demonstrated increased delta activity in schizophrenic patients. Buchsbaum (1982) has also reported increased frontal delta activity in schizophrenic patients using a different EEG topographic technique. This delta activity, which is greatest in frontal regions, may be related to findings reported by Ingvar and Franzen (1974a) in the first application of regional cerebral blood flow in psychiatric patients. Ingvar and Franzen found that

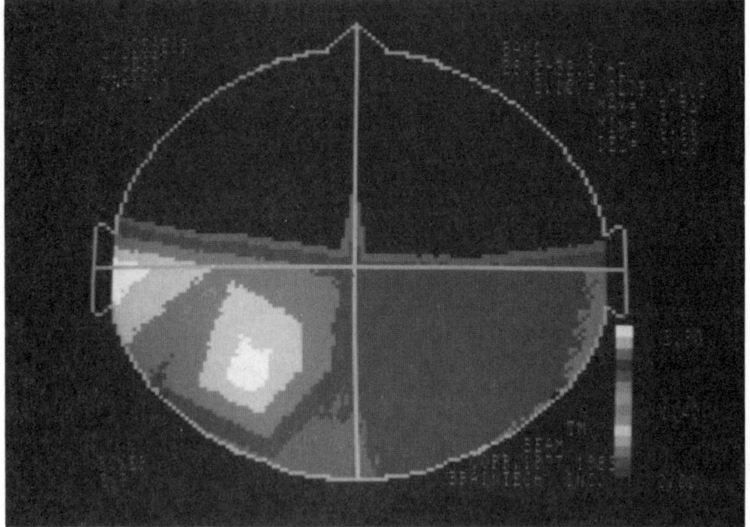

Figure 6. Significance probability map comparing fast beta activity of unmedicated schizophrenic patients with normal controls. The most marked difference is seen in the left temporal-parietal region. This figure is reprinted from a study of unmedicated schizophrenic patients (Morihisa et al. 1983a).

schizophrenic patients demonstrated a relative decrease in frontal blood flow compared to alcoholic controls. This finding, along with data from another study by Ingvar et al. (1976), which reported a correlation between mean EEG frequency and cerebral blood flow, may be relevant to recent BEAM findings. If schizophrenic patients have decreased frontal blood flow, then they could also be expected to exhibit increased delta activity that was greatest in frontal regions. Indeed, we found this pattern of increased delta activity in schizophrenic patients using BEAM. Ingvar's work suggests that schizophrenic patients have reduced neural metabolic activity in frontal regions. This early work, considered with the regional differences found in delta activity for our schizophrenic patients, suggests that the frontal lobes may be a pathologic site important to our understanding of schizophrenia. Moreover, the work presented in this volume utilizing positron emission tomography (PET) also indicates a relative reduction in

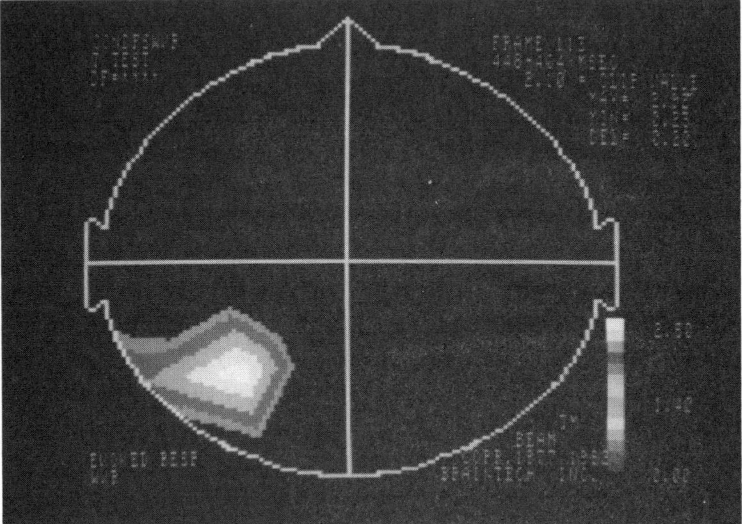

Figure 7. Significance probability map comparing the visual evoked potential of unmedicated schizophrenic patients and that of normal controls. This map shows a difference in the left parietal region at 448 msec after the flash of light and lasting over 20 msec. This figure is reprinted from a study of unmedicated schizophrenic patients (Morihisa et al. 1983a).

neural metabolic activity in the frontal cortex of schizophrenic patients. Finally, the chapter in this volume by Berman and Weinberger suggests that certain activation tests of cognition may further elaborate deficits in frontal cortical function in patients with schizophrenia.

However, the cerebral blood flow findings of Ingvar that suggested the initial hypothesis were not demonstrated in all of his patients. Furthermore, as pointed out by Prohovnik, Berman, Weinberger, and Gur, studies of regional cerebral blood flow in the resting state have a number of limitations. In addition, contradictory findings have been reported (Matthew et al. 1982 and Mubrin et al. 1982). Indeed, in this monograph, Berman, Weinberger, and Gur do not report relative reduction in frontal metabolic activity in the resting state but only paradoxically, in Weinberger's study, during cognitive activation. Together the cerebral blood flow evidence reported in this volume implicates possible frontal lobe dysfunction in schizophrenia. PET findings by Buchsbaum also indicate that patients with affective disorders demonstrate relative reduction in frontal neural metabolic activity. Hence, abnormalities of frontal lobe metabolism may not be specific to schizophrenia, but may still reflect pathophysiological sites important in our investigation of schizophrenia.

Thus, although work in brain imaging provides some encouraging convergence of findings, it has also been difficult to replicate results and to characterize physiological pathology that may be specific to certain diagnostic categories.

These contradictions and complications of interpretation emphasize that conclusions should not be drawn too quickly about the findings of brain imaging in psychiatry. It is possible that the heterogeneity of various mental disorders, as well as differences in technique and instrumentation, may contribute to difficulties in interpreting results. It is also probable that many of these findings are epiphenomena, which will interfere with the attempt to understand the processes underlying psychiatric illness. Whatever the source of such problems, they underscore the need for caution not only in applying brain-imaging techniques but also in interpreting and using their results. These techniques must be used as tools in our search for understanding disease processes. Just as we should not draw premature conclusions, however, we must also not discard tools too quickly because they do not provide elegant and unambiguous solutions. These tools are newly added to our research armamentarium and we have yet to determine how they can best be used in our clinical work. The application of brain-imaging techniques in psychiatry consists not only of conducting studies and interpreting data to generate and test hypotheses, but also of testing and refining the machines and how they are used. For now, we must follow each of the paths the new work suggests with the understanding that the road to clinical applications is often complex and filled with frustrations and surprises.

In this light, the findings of the present study suggest a further hypothesis to explore. The findings of increased posterior fast beta activity, maximal in the left parietal region, and increased beta variability, along with the augmented visual evoked potential in the parietal region, provide evidence of focal cortical irritability in this region. Although BEAM provides only two-dimensional "views" of brain electrical activity recorded from the scalp, it has better temporal resolution than the three-dimensional tomographic techniques such as PET. Using evoked potentials, electrophysiological imaging techniques can examine transient cognitive phenomena that take place in milliseconds, rather than over the 10 minutes or more required by PET scan.

Further investigation will be required to determine how these BEAM findings in the left parietal region might be related to Gur's demonstration of left hemispheric overactivation in schizophrenia. However, in this volume Buchsbaum reports abnormalities in the left parietal region in schizophrenic patients using evoked potentials. This work suggests that the left posterior quadrant, and the left parietal region in particular, may be a significant pathophysiological site in the schizophrenic process. This region is of special interest in cognitive theory and may be related to the disorders of thinking which are characteristic of schizophrenia. Furthermore, our findings are consistent with the early work of Ingvar and Franzen (1974b), who reported that blood flow increases in post-central temporal-occipital and parietal regions were associated with symptoms of disturbed cognition. Additional research will be required to confirm and further elaborate this association.

CONCLUSION

We have seen how by using the new computerized brain-imaging techniques of regional cerebral blood flow (rCBF), positron emission tomography (PET), and brain electrical activity mapping (BEAM), we can examine the metabolism and electrophysiology of the normal and pathological brain. We have reported some of the most recent findings, which indicate some patterns that may help us understand mental illness and suggest new avenues of investigation. However, we have also detailed some of the limitations inherent in the use of brain-imaging techniques to understand mental processes. All these points may help the reader assimilate brain-imaging studies of psychiatric disorders. Not only are we dependent on technological developments, but we also must expect to travel down false paths and pursue frustrating leads in the investigation of mental illness as we continue the dynamic process of fitting our technical capability to our clinical interests. These different approaches do not represent competing methods but rather complementary views of brain function. In fact, it is through applying them in concert that we may help solve some of the puzzles of mental illness. In this chapter, the findings from different techniques have been considered together to look for meaningful patterns. Instead of conclusions, we hope the reader has been left with new hypotheses to explore.

References

American Psychiatric Association: Diagnostic and Statistical Manual of Mental Disorders, 3rd ed. Washington, DC, American Psychiatric Association, 1980

Berger H: Uber das elektrenkephalogramm des Menschen I. Arch Psychiatr Nervenkr 87:527–571, 1929

Buchsbaum MS, Cappelletti J, Coppola R, et al: New methods to determine the CNS effects of antigeriatric compounds: EEG topography and glucose use. Drug Development Research 2:489–496, 1982

Dement WC, Fisher C: Experimental interference with the sleep cycle. Canadian Psychiatric Association Journal 8:400–405, 1963

Duffy FH, Burchfiel JL, Lombroso CT: Brain electrical activity mapping (BEAM): a method for extending the clinical utility of EEG and evoked potential data. Ann Neurol 5:309–332, 1979

Duffy FH, Bartels PH, Burchfiel JL: Significance probability mapping: an aid in the topographic analysis of brain electrical activity. Electroencephalogr Clin Neurophysiol 51:455–462, 1981

Gershon ES, Buchsbaum MS: A genetic study of average evoked response augmentation/reduction in affective disorders, in Psychopathology and Brain Dysfunction. Edited by Shagass C, Gershon S, Friedhoff AJ. New York, Raven Press, 1977

Gillin J, Post R, Wyatt RJ, et al: Infusion of threodihydroxyphenylserine (DOPS) and 5-hydroxytryptophan (5HTP) during human sleep. Sleep Research 1:45, 1972

Ingvar DH, Franzen G: Abnormalities of cerebral blood flow distribution in patients with chronic schizophrenia. Acta Psychiatr Scand 50:425–462, 1974a

Ingvar DH, Franzen G: Distribution of cerebral activity in chronic schizophrenia. Lancet 2:1484–1486, 1974b

Ingvar DH, Sjolund B, Ardo A: Correlation between dominant EEG frequency, cerebral oxygen uptake and blood flow. Electroencephalogr Clin Neurophysiol 41:268–276, 1976

Itil TM, Saleut B, Davis S: EEG findings in chronic schizophrenics based on digital computer period analysis and analog power spectra. Biol Psychiatry 5:1–13, 1972

Kupfer DH, Foster FG, Detre TP: Sleep continuity changes in depression. Diseases of the Nervous System 34:192–195, 1973

Matthew RJ, Duncan GC, Weinman ML, et al: Regional cerebral blood flow in schizophrenia. Arch Gen Psychiatry 39:1121–1124, 1982

Morihisa JM, Duffy FH, Wyatt RJ: Topographic analysis of computer processed electroencephalography in schizophrenia, in Biological Markers in Psychiatry and Neurology. Edited by Usdin E, Hanin J. New York, Pergamon Press, 1982

Morihisa JM, Duffy FH, Wyatt RJ: Brain electrical activity mapping (BEAM) in schizophrenic patients. Arch Gen Psychiatry 40:719–728, 1983a

Morihisa JM, Duffy FH, Mendelson WB, et al: The use of brain electrical activity mapping (BEAM) as an exploratory technique to delineate regional differences between schizophrenic patients and control subjects, in Laterality and Psychopathology. Edited by Flor-Henry P, Gruzelier J. New York, Elsevier, 1983b

Mubrin A, Knezvic S, Koretic D, et al: Regional cerebral blood flow patterns in schizophrenic patients. Regional Cerebral Blood Flow Bulletin 3:43–46, 1982

Rechtschaffen A, Schulsinger F, Mednick SA: Schizophrenia and physiological indices of dreaming. Arch Gen Psychiatry 10:89–93, 1964

Shagass C, Roemer RA, Straumanis J, et al: Temporal variability of somatosensory, visual and auditory evoked potentials in schizophrenia. Arch Gen Psychiatry 36:1341–1351, 1979

Shagass C, Roemer R, Staumanis J, et al: Topography of sensory evoked potentials in depressive disorders. Biol Psychiatry 15:183–207, 1980

Spitzer RL, Endicott J, Robins E: Research Diagnostic Criteria for a Selected Group of Functional Disorders, 3rd ed. New York, Biometrics Research Division, New York State Psychiatric Institute, 1977

Stevens JR, Livermore A: Telemetered EEG in schizophrenia: spectral analysis during abnormal behavior episodes. J Neurol Neurosurg Psychiatry 45:385–395, 1982

Tukey J: Exploratory Data Analysis. Reading, MA, Addison-Wesley, 1977